Sparky Fights Back

Sparky Fights Back

A Little Dog's Big Battle Against Cancer

Josée Clerens and John Clifton

Second printing 2005

Additional copies and information:
Visit our web site at www.SparkyFightsBack.com for further information,
continuously updated resources on animal cancer, and to order additional
copies of this book.

A substantial portion of the proceeds from the sale of this book will go to the
Animal Cancer Foundation, New York, NY (www.acfoundation.org).

ATTENTION CORPORATIONS, UNIVERSITIES, COLLEGES, AND
PROFESSIONAL AND CHARITABLE ORGANIZATIONS: Quantity
discounts are available on bulk purchases of this book for educational and
gift purposes, or as premiums in fundraising efforts. Inquiries should be
addressed to Foley Square Books, P. O. Box 20548, Park West Station, New
York, NY 10025; VOICE: 212-724-1578 FAX: 775-514-1760

ISBN 0-9760846-0-0

LCCN 2004113106

Hope is part of the human spirit to endure and give a miracle a chance to happen.

—Jerome Groopman, *The Anatomy of Hope* [2004]

Authors' Note

This book is written in the first person singular, even though it was a close collaboration of two people, neither of whom is single; in fact they are a married couple—happily plural. For reasons of style and clarity, however, the story is told in the voice of Josée, the wife.

Also, please note that many of the medical professionals included here have since moved to other institutions and facilities.

—J.C. & J.C.

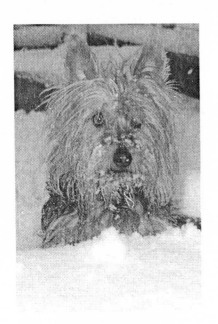
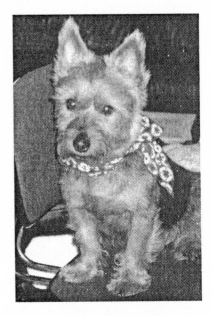

Before treatment
(In the snow)

During treatment
(Showing hair loss)

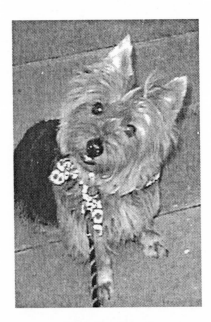

After treatment

Contents

Acknowledgments

When your pet is diagnosed with cancer, you need all the help you can get. So many people helped us throughout the experience of fighting Sparky's disease and putting this book together, it's impossible to list them all. It seemed like everyone—neighbors, close friends and fleeting acquaintances alike—wanted to help, to contribute in some way in alleviating our pain. Many of them appear in the book, so we won't name them here. But we want to express our gratitude to all. The members of the veterinary community and animal medical specialists who treated Sparky seemed to go far beyond the mere dispensing of medical treatment, generously offering their sincere concern and advice. In this regard, we especially thank Dr. Gerald Post, Dr. Bonnie Brown, and Dr. Sheri Siegel.

Our editor, Danelle McCafferty, simply was the best. She helped us shape and focus the narrative, and gave us so many good suggestions (*most* of which we followed!). Samantha Schmidt not only wrote the foreword, but unknowingly sparked the idea for the book. It was at her request that we wrote an article for the newsletter of the Animal Cancer Foundation. The response from that brief account of Sparky's illness led to the writing of the book itself. Also, special thanks to Laurie Kaplan for her professional advice, and Aberjhani for editing an early version of the manuscript.

Lastly, we wish to thank all the dog owners who have visited our website, most of them seeking help for their own cancer-stricken pets. Many have taken the time to write us, sharing their experiences. They have shown that there is a strong need for a book such as this, further encouraging us to take on the task of writing it. We wish them luck, and hope that these pages offer some measure of comfort and hope.

Foreword

by Samantha J. Schmidt

I am a big believer in the tasteful presentation of medical matters. I have never liked ads that try to make your gut roll with horror and your heart ache with pity. People can understand a need without having their reactions painfully manipulated. This is one reason why Sparky's story impressed me. It simply lets the facts speak for themselves. Here you will see the roller coaster of emotions that the owner of a pet with cancer goes through. You'll see the choices the owner is faced with. You'll see the insecurity that comes with making decisions about your animal's care. And you will see the need for reliable, sound information.

Serving as the Director of the Animal Cancer Foundation has been both rewarding and painful. I speak to people daily who are navigating through the complex emotions and logistics that go along with discovering their pet has cancer: "I didn't even know dogs and cats got cancer." "I didn't know there were treatments for animals with cancer." "I can't lose my best friend." "I don't have the money for treatments for my pet." These are common daily remarks from people who call ACF.

I came to ACF quite by chance. I had learned of its existence when my Great Dane, Beau, was diagnosed with lymphoma. Beau succumbed to complications from the disease within one month at 8 ½ years old. I did not meet Dr. Gerald S. Post, ACF's founder, until two years after Beau passed away. I had heard that he was the man with the answers and the direct, no-beating-around-the-bush approach. He was looking for someone to organize a Foundation event. He wanted to educate people about ACF's work. I thought "What an easy sell!" I still think that today.

Clearly the need is there. People need information, direction and options; they want to combat animal cancer so it cannot take another pet. And later I learned the extra benefit— that by studying pets with cancer we can learn valuable information about human cancer, treatments, and even preventative measures. It seems so simple once it is pointed out: Our animals live with us, in our environments. They breathe the same air and share the same nutritional base. Their physical reactions are remarkably similar to ours. I realized that ACF was in a position to expose these ideas, and develop studies based upon these concepts. Exactly what it is doing today.

Sparky's story is a happy one. *Sparky Fights Back* underlines the need for the Animal Cancer Foundation. It holds important lessons for anyone whose life has been touched by cancer—whether human or animal. Cancer is a harsh reality of our time. We need to use *every resource we have* to try and delete it as an everyday word. The Animal Cancer Foundation continues to impact cancer through research, education and prevention. ACF and Sparky give owners hope, which is a good place to start.

The Alarm

"It's probably lymphoma," said Dr. Bonnie Brown, of Animal General in New York City. She had just finished examining Sparky, our six-year-old Australian terrier. About a week earlier we had noticed lumps on his throat, little swellings about the size of grapes. More alarming, he had lost his appetite. My husband, John, suspected swollen glands and had called the vet's office. The young woman who answered the phone said we should watch for any further developments, and if Sparky didn't get better to call back.

We hadn't been that concerned. Just about every problem we'd ever had with Sparky could be traced back to his insistence on picking up all kinds of debris off the sidewalk. A discarded French fry, piece of bagel, or tossed bone too often found its way into his mouth. He couldn't stop himself—food was Sparky's main interest in life. "Drop it" was a command we had to use constantly. He would obey at once, and then instantly pick up the item again. It was maddening—a small dog, close to the ground, and lightning quick.

Although we watched him closely all the time he was outside, he was too clever for us. Not only on the sidewalks, but in the park as well. Like many other New Yorkers, John took his dog to the park nearly every day, an excursion both enjoyed equally. That, plus two more outings a day, held untold opportunities for Sparky to exploit.

And exploit them he did. His medical records were filled with stomach ailments, tapeworms, rashes, and other adverse reactions caused by his nasty habit of snatching up foreign matter. Just a year earlier, he had had to have surgery to remove a twig lodged in his throat. So here again, surely, was yet another similar episode, I thought. It just couldn't be cancer. Our lively, ebullient little terrier had cancer? Impossible.

Dr. Brown, as bonny as her name and with a natural affinity for animals—certainly for our Sparky— said she hoped it wasn't lymphoma, that there was a chance it could be something else. The only way to be certain was to perform a biopsy. All right; we'd do that. John asked her what the chances were for a dog with lymphoma. She said the disease was "treatable but not curable."

John looked crestfallen. Dr. Brown began to use some serious-sounding terms: bone-marrow aspiration, lymph node excision, histopathology, cytology, ultrasound, and I don't remember what else. Nevertheless, I felt confident none of that would be necessary. Dr. Brown took Sparky into another room to take some tissue and blood samples. We waited silently. She returned with him a short while later.

"We'll have the results late tomorrow," she said. "There's a chance it may be something benign; we'll see. I'll call you tomorrow evening."

We hoped and prayed it would turn out to be something benign. It *might* not be lymphoma. There was at least a *chance*.

We put Sparky's leash on him, paid our bill at the front desk, and left Animal General. Dr. Brown had seemed warmly sympathetic and thoroughly competent. But we still couldn't believe she could be right.

"Do you think we should get another opinion?" John asked.

"Who from?" I wondered. The whole thing seemed so scary. We were both afraid of making a mistake at this point. We needed to know as much as we could. Thousands of uncertainties bounced around in my mind. Was it really lymphoma? How long would we have Sparky before—before *what*? We walked on a bit, neither of us speaking. Sparky, oblivious and unconcerned, meandered along with us, frequently pulling over for the occasional exploratory sniff of some particular attraction or other. Which he would then instantly mark, by lifting his leg.

Another dog owner in our building had told John about a big veterinary hospital across town. "Maybe we should go there," John said, rather tentatively. "They're supposed to be the best." He wasn't himself; I could see that. John's not the type to lose his head in an emergency. Yet here he was, seeming stunned and bewildered by it all.

"All right. Let's get the number and we'll call them tomorrow," I said.

Our apartment was only a block away from Animal General, but that walk home held enough thoughts and feelings to fill a mile. We would never forget that day—August 8, 2000.

The next day we made the appointment at the prestigious Animal Medical Center on East 62nd Street in Manhattan. John put Sparky in his Sherpa bag, a special container for small animals resembling a locker bag with see-through mesh sides. We took the 86th Street crosstown bus. After two stops, David, an associate of John's and fellow teacher at Columbia Grammar and Prep School, boarded the bus and spotted us sitting there with this luggage on our laps.

We told David where we were going and why. He knew Sparky. In fact, just about everyone at the school knew Sparky; he had accompanied John there during many of my husband's off-hours work in his computer lab.

David's face was sympathetic. "Well, I hope it comes out all right," he said. "Maybe it's just a false alarm."

John opened the zipper of the Sherpa bag, and Sparky stuck out his head. Immediately, people on the bus reacted to Sparky's "high cute factor," as one book described the attraction certain dogs generate. Just by being himself, he was irresistible. Even now, confined in a bag and threatened by a serious illness, he remained his remarkable self.

Which is to say, strikingly unusual. And, even in "sophisticated" New York, most people aren't familiar with the breed. In terms of coloring, there are two types of Australian terriers. One is called "red," meaning that the dog's color is uniformly reddish-golden. The second type, Sparky's, is called "blue and tan"—by far the better known. Blue and tans have reddish-golden heads, manes, legs, and feet. Their necks, backs and the tops of their tails are mostly blackish. If you separate the hairs of the blackish part, you see where the "blue" comes in. The skin underneath has a decidedly bluish cast. Some people at first mistake an Aussie for a large Yorkshire terrier (Sparky typically weighs about eighteen to twenty pounds). But Aussies are nothing like Yorkies in characteristics or temperament. And, for that matter, Sparky is like no other dog—including other Aussies.

Beyond Sparky's distinct appearance, people are immediately taken with his singular personality. Sparky doesn't fuss over people as many dogs do. No putting his paws on someone's legs, tail wagging, or face licking of just-met humans for him. No, Sparky's approach is not that of your typical "cute dog." Sparky will stare at a person, his deep, dark eyes peering from behind his silky top-knot. He doesn't outwardly greet someone unless he knows them, and knows them well. Sparky studies, evaluates, and makes a serious attempt to figure out what the person is all about.

When you speak to Sparky, he listens. I mean, he really *listens*. His head cocks from one side to the other, while his brain seems to work at full capacity deciphering the meaning of your words. And somehow, *somehow*, he speaks back. Call it telepathy or voodoo, you understand, perhaps by the look in his eyes, what he is trying to convey.

The bus crossed through Central Park and reached the East Side. We came to our stop. "Good luck," David said, as we stepped off.

We transferred to the downtown bus on York Avenue. After getting off at 62nd Street, we walked east a short block to the Animal Medical Center. The facility occupies several floors, practically like a human hospital. It has an entire oncology *department*—very impressive. We sat in the huge waiting room, which was filled with a variety of animals needing attention, accompanied by their anxious human companions. Our turn finally came.

Two very young female vets—one of them may have been an intern—greeted us and took us to one of the examination rooms. On the way, I was thinking, hoping, that we would soon be told that Dr. Brown was in error. There was a *chance*. Maybe...maybe... The one we thought to be the veterinarian spoke first. "What can we do for you today?"

"We came for a second opinion," John told her. "He's got these lumps on his throat, and we took him to our regular vet yesterday. She said it might be lymphoma. She took a biopsy, but we haven't gotten the results yet."

"Let's have a look."

John lifted Sparky up onto her table.

"What's his name?" she asked brightly—a little *too* brightly, I thought.

"Sparky."

She turned to the dog. "Okay, Sparky."

She ran her hands under his chin and over his body, ending up with the hind legs. She listened with her stethoscope, then took his temperature with a rectal thermometer. It all seemed quite routine, and she smiled all through it. Then she turned to us. The whole room, and everything and everyone in it, froze for a second—a very long second. My heart seemed to stop beating. I didn't look at John, perhaps because I feared he was as petrified as I was.

"Based on what I'm seeing here, I expect the biopsy to show lymphoma."

John clasped my hand. I burst into tears. We had spent all this time only to hear Dr. Brown's opinion confirmed! The one we assumed to be the intern offered what she must have thought was consolation: "With proper treatment, Sparky might even live ten to twelve months."

"But he's only six years old," John protested. "Isn't that too young to get cancer?"

"No, that's about right for these guys, five, six—pretty typical."

All I could think was I wanted to get out of there and take Sparky home.

"Some of these guys really rally, and live as long as two years," she said by way of encouragement.

"Well, thank you," said John, forcing politeness.

Devastated, we paid the bill and headed home. I couldn't stop crying. By some quirky coincidence, David happened to be on the 86th Street cross-town bus again.

"What's the outcome?" he asked. But he had certainly already guessed, just by looking at us.

"They came up with the same opinion," John told him. Sparky's adorable face peeked out the top of the Sherpa bag, and John lightly rested on his hand on our Aussie's head.

That evening, Dr. Brown called. John answered the phone.

"Hi, Dr. Brown." John listened for a moment.

I could tell from his voice that the news wasn't good. I was cooking dinner and came out of the kitchen to listen.

"It's lymphosarcoma," he said to me, momentarily covering the receiver. "Is that the same thing as lymphoma?" he asked Dr. Brown. He nodded to me, indicating that it was. "There can't be any mistake?" he asked the doctor. He looked at me and shook his head. That was the moment I realized that there would be no hope of any other diagnosis. Sparky had cancer. Unquestionably. I tried to concentrate on the conversation. Dr. Brown was recommending that we start chemotherapy treatments immediately.

"We need to go to an oncologist," John whispered to me, then spoke into the phone. "We went over to Animal Medical Center today. Perhaps we should take him there for the treatments." He paused. Then to me: "She says that would be okay, but there's an oncologist at Animal Medical. Dr. Post." He wrote the name down.

He listened for a little, then asked Dr. Brown if she would hold on for a minute. He put the phone on hold.

"She says that Animal General has an excellent oncologist named Dr. Gerald Post. He comes in once a week. She *highly* recommends him." John, perhaps still under the influence of the Animal Medical Center's impressive facility and full oncology staff, again wondered whether it wouldn't be better to take Sparky there.

"Well, I trust Dr. Brown." I was going mostly on instinct, but I did give weight to her recommendation. "What do you think?"

"Dr. Brown says that there's no one better in the field. You think we should go with him?"

"Well," I ventured, "it would be closer—and we can always change if we want."

John took the phone off hold and returned to Dr. Brown. "What day does Dr. Post come in?"

Sometimes in life a decision is made—for better or worse— that affects one so profoundly that it makes all the difference subsequently. Our choosing to go with Dr. Post was one of those decisions.

John continued on the telephone with Dr. Brown: Dr. Post only came in on Wednesday evenings. Dr. Brown arranged an appointment for us to see him the following Wednesday. Meanwhile, she explained that she wanted to do further tests, to take samples and see if the cancer had spread to the liver or any other organs. She would make up an estimate of what had to be done.

"Okay, I'll stop by tomorrow and pick it up. And thank you, Doctor." John hung up the receiver.

I told myself to calm down. After all, Sparky was just a dog. He wasn't our child. But we had no children. He *was* our child. "Keep a sense of proportion, Josée!" I urged myself. Sure, this was going to be tough, but keep a sense of proportion. I went on inwardly in this way—blah, blah, blah. None of it worked. I returned to the kitchen and went through the motions of making dinner.

John went in the next day to sign an estimate for a list of procedures Sparky would receive: lymph node excision; anesthesia and medications; Oxymorphone, and others. Then there were "Therapeutic Professional Services": fluids, catheter, etc. The estimate also totaled in the cytology and bone marrow aspiration she had already performed. He glanced at the bottom line. The "low amount" was $924 and the "high amount" $1,004. There is such a thing as veterinary insurance, but we didn't have any. This was going to be way over our budget. But somehow it didn't matter to me. Ordinarily I watch every penny, look for every bargain, cut out those endless coupons, resist shopping sprees. But this was for *Sparky*! I just didn't give a damn about the money.

A few days later on August 15, we took Sparky in at 9:00 A.M. for the surgery and tests. We checked in at the front desk. Soon, Dr. Brown appeared and took Sparky out of John's arms.

"Hi, Sparky," she said warmly, and seemed to cuddle our little boy in affectionate arms. "I won't be here this evening when you come back for him. He'll have to remain for several hours after the procedures. I'll leave you a note and we can talk tomorrow if there are any questions."

Dr. Brown turned to leave with our little terrier.

John called "Bye, Sparky" as he was carried away.

"Bye, Sweetheart!" I echoed.

Dr. Brown turned and carried Sparky down a long, narrow hallway to the rear of the facility. John and I stood there watching them retreat into the distance. Sparky wasn't struggling or squirming in her arms. He seemed entirely cooperative, but then, who can say what went on inside his mind? He rarely had been out of our care since we got him. He had always been a *good* dog. There was that independent streak of his, of course, about a mile wide. But when it counted, he could pull himself together and cooperate. That's called *trust*: "I don't like this one bit. I'd rather pull loose and cut out of here. I'd like to put up a big stink about the whole thing! But I won't. I'm doing it for *you*."

The door at the end of the corridor opened, then closed, and Sparky and the doctor were gone. John and I grasped each other's hand. There would be an empty spot in our hearts till he was back with us again.

That evening, I wasn't up to cooking. We opted for a bite in a neighborhood restaurant. I can't remember that meal at all, what we ate, or what we said. There was nothing we could do now but wait. It was all out of our hands. We felt helpless. At least we would get Sparky back later that evening.

On the way to the restaurant we passed by Animal General.

"I wonder how our little guy is doing," I said.

"Maybe we can take a peek," John suggested.

The operating room is at the far rear of the building, which is on the corner of 87th Street and Columbus Avenue. The entrance is on Columbus, and the 87th Street side is lined with large plate glass windows. We knew that the last was the window of the operating room. A huge window blind prevented passers-by from looking inside, but there was a narrow gap at the edge of the glass that the blind didn't cover. John tried to peek through. He couldn't see much, but he did make out the cage with Sparky in it.

"Is he sleeping?" I asked.

"No. He's standing up. Pacing a little bit."

"He doesn't like it."

"You're right."

"Don't let him see you." That would be disastrous, I thought—for him to see us and not be able to get out of there.

"Don't worry," John said. "He can't smell us, and he won't recognize much through this little crack."

Sparky in a cage. An image I found hard to take. It is said that animals accept whatever happens—that they can't imagine a reality other than the here and now. And so they kind of go with the flow of events. But that doesn't mean they like it. And Sparky doesn't like to be locked up. Except for when he was neutered, shortly after we purchased him, Sparky had never been separated from us. We plan vacations so that he might be part of them. Kennels are out of the question. If it's impractical to take him along, well then, we won't go. We never consider this a hardship or a nuisance; it's simply our choice.

After dinner we went to pick up Sparky. A female attendant carried him out from the operating room down that long hallway to meet us. Sparky, eager to give us a proper greeting, tried to wriggle out of the attendant's arms. She put him onto the floor and he hit the ground running. He raced toward us. It was pure delight; he jumped back and forth from John to me, his head tucked down between his shoulders, his ears laid back, and his docked little tail vibrating so fast it blurred. There were bandages on his rear leg and elsewhere, as I recall. The attendant gave us some medications and instructions with a hand-written report from the doctor:

8/15/00

Mr. And Mrs. Clifton,

Sparky did very well in surgery today. We took a small wedge of tissue from the lymph node in his left hind leg for biopsy and we did a bone marrow aspirate from his right hip. I put a "stat" on the biopsy and hope we'll have it back for your appointment with Dr. Post tomorrow. The stitches behind his left knee will need to come out in 10-14 days.

Sparky was a great patient today—we'll see you and him tomorrow. Thank you—

Dr. Brown

Sparky can eat a small meal <u>later</u> this evening.

We took Sparky home. That night, he slept like a baby, which is more than I can say for John and me.

Buying Time

———————✹———————

Our first appointment with the oncologist was scheduled for the following evening. We took Sparky in to Animal General and told Mary, the receptionist, that we had an appointment with Dr. Post. "Oh, yes," she said, "he's got a very good track record. He also tells it like it is."

We took a seat and waited. Dr. Brown came out briefly to check with us about everything. She said hi to Sparky, who was sitting between John and me, and gave him a kiss on the top of his head. She reviewed what she'd written in her report and reminded us about our appointment the next morning. Sparky would undergo further examination using ultrasound. She said they would have to shave his belly for this and to plan on leaving him there for the day. Sparky wasn't going to be exactly thrilled about this—and neither was I.

Dr. Brown then left, and soon afterward, we met Dr. Post. He came into the waiting room and looked at us. "Sparky?" he asked.

"Yes," we said, and rose to follow him to an examination room. He was a friendly looking fellow probably in his late thirties with a slight build, short hair, and stubbly beard.

Dr. Post checked Sparky's vital signs. "Here's what to expect," he said. "With no treatment, he'll live about a month. With chemotherapy he'll probably survive twelve, maybe

fourteen months. That's what you can *expect*. As far as a cure—
well, there's no way I can promise anything."

"Twelve to fourteen months"—pretty much what the
Animal Medical vet had told us. That hopeless, fatalistic feeling
returned, momentarily invading my thoughts. Still, Dr. Post's
words painted a picture that was at least paradoxical—bleak,
but not without a scintilla of hope. "After all," we would tell
each other later, "he didn't *rule out* a cure. That scintilla, that
tiny grain of *possibility* of a cure, was to carry us through many
a difficult and discouraging time.

Sparky, the doctor told us, would go into remission
rather quickly—in a week or two. Dogs, it seems, have a much
more immediate reaction to the chemo than humans. John had
been doing some research the past few days on the Internet.
Humans with "non-Hodgkins lymphoma" follow a different
scenario than canines. Of humans who contract the disease,
about half go into remission. Of this half, most all remain in
remission, or survive. With dogs, virtually all go into
remission, but hardly any remain in remission indefinitely.
Most die after a year.

A dog in remission typically leads a relatively normal,
active life. The chemo is certainly not without side-effects, but
they are less severe and persistent than with humans. Sparky
would have a bad day here and there, but otherwise would
lead a normal dog's life.

Dr. Post went over all the details of the treatment
protocol. It would last for one year. The year of chemotherapy
treatments would initially be a week apart, then two, then

monthly, then at two-month intervals. A full year of treatments—that seemed a lot, I thought.

He estimated the cost of the treatments at $7,000. With extras and other treatments, it would actually come to $12,000 by the end of the year. But Sparky had given us so much. He had rejuvenated our life and filled our every day with joy. The least *we* could give him in return was another year of life. And so we embarked upon this pay-as-you-go journey, buying life a day at a time. It would be worth the fare, no matter what.

Sparky would receive his first chemotherapy treatment immediately. Dr. Post left the tiny exam room to fetch the chemicals and paraphernalia. Sparky tried to jump off the stainless steel table. John held him until the doctor returned with a nurse to assist with the procedure.

Sparky would receive Vincristine, a chemical that is also used in human chemotherapy. In fact, we would learn, Sparky would receive the exact same chemicals that a human cancer victim would get—Vincristine, Elspar ("Asparaginase"), Cytoxan and Adriamycin. The Vincristine was injected into his right hind leg, since the recent biopsy incision had been made on the left one. The nurse and the doctor, standing on opposite sides of the table, rolled Sparky onto his side. The nurse's job was to pin him down and keep him still while the doctor administered the chemical through a catheter. Dr. Post carefully measured the liquid, then slowly and methodically controlled its flow into Sparky's vein.

John bent down and spoke to Sparky in his best falsetto. We had learned, somewhere along the line, that speaking in a high, soft tone is calming to dogs. Sparky was frightened, but for the most part lay motionless for the procedure. "Still...still..." John would chant, "Good still..."

Sparky knew the word and what it meant, from previous training. We were so proud of him. It was no small thing for him to be pinned down that way. He must have felt helpless and frightened. His pleading eyes looked directly into my husband's, as if to ask, "What's going on? What are they doing to me?" Though the procedure lasted only a few minutes, it seemed to take forever. Sparky never put up a fuss. What a good little guy, I thought. Then, suddenly it was done. Dr. Post removed the needle, then cleaned and bandaged the wound. The nurse released his pressure, and Sparky righted himself onto all fours.

We thanked Dr. Post and left the exam room to make an appointment for the next visit with him, and for several succeeding weeks as well. Mary handed John some Prednisone tablets, to counter side effects of the Vincristine, with dosage instructions. John wrote out a check. We said good night and took Sparky, wearing his new bandage, home. One of our neighbors saw us approaching the main entrance of our building and inquired about Sparky. Practically everyone in our entire complex of 266 apartments seemed to know Sparky. Word of his disease had already gotten around. We told her he had just had his first chemo treatment.

"Brave little boy," she said. Some people think New Yorkers aren't very friendly. Somewhere they have gotten the impression that we don't care about—or even know—our neighbors. Untrue. Here was a neighbor, like *hundreds* of others, showing great concern over a little *dog*! It's hard to imagine that happening any place *but* New York.

She crouched down to pet Sparky. He didn't recoil. First of all, he had known her for a long time. Second, she was *not* a little kid. It was reassuring to know that Sparky didn't reject *everybody*.

Sparky is indeed indifferent to most people—to strangers certainly—as I've mentioned. When he meets a new person they often extend their hand to let him sniff it, a common practice, especially among dog owners. Sparky looks at the hand just long enough to see if there is a treat in it. Children frighten him; toddlers in particular he views as a threat. Nothing upsets him more than a toddler veering in his direction and squealing, "A puppy! A puppy!" He will catch sight of them long before they notice him and bark a warning not to come closer, all the while keeping a watchful eye on the advancing menace. Because of his small size and overall cuddly appearance, this intense staring is nearly every time misinterpreted by the parent, or child, or both, as an invitation to a closer acquaintance. Often the toddler will lunge forward, arms outstretched and emitting high-pitched shrieks of delight only to stop dead, aghast at Sparky's furious barking.

Once this very scene played out in a large outlet store in Vermont. The child was a sweet-looking little girl who burst into tears at Sparky's reaction. So John picked Sparky up and urged the little girl to pet him—Sparky didn't bite, never had, children or anyone else—and off the ground, on John's arm, somehow whatever threat these children posed disappeared.

Also, John didn't want the little girl to grow up with a fear of all dogs because of one rude Australian terrier.

We had discovered earlier—quite by accident—that our dog's behavior toward strangers, old as well as young, was completely different when he was off the ground. We had been shopping once in a pet supply store and Sparky was riding around in a shopping cart. He seemed delighted to be wheeled around like a canine potentate among all these attractive doggie items and treats with their highly agreeable aromas. At one point, a very nice little boy came up to him and started to pet him. To our amazement, Sparky was quite congenial, totally devoid of his usual anti-child defenses. We thought the reason was that the boy had treated him so gently. But after subsequent observations we put two and two together: he was very nice to *everyone*, so long as he was on their level—in a chair, on a bench, or cradled in our arms.

Where his fear originally came from we haven't a clue. And, while it has diminished over the years, it hasn't gone away. Even if a child is safely ensconced in a stroller, Sparky will cast a wary eye on it and keep it there until the stroller and its occupant are well out of sight.

The first time we noticed this was when he was still a puppy and we were watching *Forrest Gump* on video. There is a scene in that movie when Forrest is a small child and walks with braces on his legs. His mother urges him to walk—no, run. "Run, Forrest, run!" she shouts, and the boy does. It was at that point our newly acquired terrier started barking passionately at the screen and Forrest, going so far as to check behind the TV to make sure this running menace wasn't coming into the room. John and I were very entertained by this display and had to roll the tape back a bit to see the part we'd missed, as well as to see if he would do it again. But, to our disappointment, he didn't repeat his performance. Sparky is nothing if not logical. He figured out quickly that there was no point in looking behind the set—or in looking at the screen for that matter. Whatever was going on there had no scent and never spilled beyond its borders. Regardless of how loud the noise or furious the shouting, it was all much ado about nothing as far as he was concerned. He had been fooled once; he wasn't going to be fooled again!

Our neighbor wished us good luck and continued on her way. We continued home. John removed the Band-Aid from Sparky's hind leg where he had received the injection and I fixed his dinner. That night, John went to his computer and did a search for the four chemicals that Sparky would receive. Being a computer teacher, he's very adept at finding information on the Internet. He had already started a collection of printouts from web pages concerning all sorts of information on lymphoma and other related matters. The page on Vincristine included such information as:

WHAT ARE THE POSSIBLE SIDE EFFECTS?

- *Hair loss*
- *Nausea/Vomiting*
- *Numbness and tingling in the feet and hands*
- *Jaw pain*

This wasn't exactly going to be a smooth ride, I thought. Of course, the information was intended for humans, not dogs. Still, we had read about many similarities in the way humans and animals are affected by cancer treatment.

The next day John took Sparky in for his ultrasound. Once again, he had to leave him there and drop by later to pick him up. The purpose, Dr. Brown explained, was to see if the cancer had spread to any of his internal organs. The one it would most likely affect was the liver. We prayed that the disease had been caught early and hadn't metastasized. If it had spread to his liver or stomach, the situation would be very bad. I think John and I both, while waiting for the results, added a few gray hairs that day.

That evening, Dr. Brown called. She had finished the procedure and said we could come get Sparky. The ultrasound showed no metastasis. The cancer hadn't spread outside his lymphatic system. John and I, filled with gratitude, gave each other a hug. John went to Animal General and brought Sparky home.

Sparky slept soundly that night. However, the next morning he didn't keep his breakfast down. This was followed by diarrhea and weakness. It was as if he had been poisoned. And, in a way, he had. He had always been so healthy, barring the typical maladies that all dogs experience. Now he was so weak he didn't resemble himself.

John took him out that morning for his morning walk, but only as far as the curb in front of our building. Usually they might walk several blocks, but not this morning. On the way back home, they came upon the two steps that rise up from the sidewalk level to the walkway leading to the main entrance. Sparky, barely hobbling along, hesitated at the first step. He looked up at John.

"What's the matter, Sparky? C'mon, let's go," John said, gently prompting him to climb up.

But Sparky put one paw up onto the first step and froze, then looked up pathetically at John.

"What is it?" John asked. Sparky just wasn't moving. John was puzzled. Then it dawned on him. The dog was simply too weak. "That's okay; I'll pick-im-up." Sparky understood "pick-im-up" as a single word, one among the hundreds he knew (yes, *hundreds*). He withdrew his paw and waited to be picked up. John lifted Sparky into his arms and carried him the rest of the way home. When I saw them coming into the apartment that way I was a little alarmed. John explained what had transpired. I felt so helpless. Sparky had always been so lively and energetic. The poor thing, why did this have to happen? Why our Sparky? I had had a bout with lung cancer many years before. John was currently dealing with prostate cancer. Wasn't that enough for one little family? Not our dog, too!

There is a small public plaza surrounding our apartment building, with trees, benches, and a play area for young children. To conserve Sparky's energy, which we now realized had been drained by the fight his body had to put up against both the disease and its treatment, John stopped taking him for his daily romp in Central Park. Now, his outings were limited to short walks up the block and sitting with one of us in our little plaza.

A few days later, John was sitting in the plaza with Sparky on his lap when Natalie, a neighbor, entered with her dog Scruffy and went over to John. Natalie was a young African-American woman who lived with her mother, a few floors up from us. Her mother, Joan, was undergoing chemotherapy for inoperable lung cancer. They knew about Sparky, and John filled Natalie in on the latest news. Natalie told John that her mother had been taking noni juice. She said that it was supposed to have very beneficial effects against cancer.

John was curious. "Where can you get it?"

"In the health food stores, but it's about forty dollars a bottle. The best stuff, though, comes from the islands. I know people there who grow it and send it up here fresh. I can't always get the fresh stuff, but I get it when I can."

By "the islands" she meant Puerto Rico, or that part of the world. Noni is actually native to Tahiti. John asked her if he could try some. She said she would bring him a jar soon. It certainly sounded interesting. John looked up noni juice on the Internet. There were all sorts of claims that it had cured people's cancer and quite a few other ailments. It seemed like it was all hype, but who knew for sure? There could be something to it.

That night, Sparky wouldn't eat his dinner. This was a shock because he was a dog who lived for food. Of course, all dogs are pretty much food-oriented, but Sparky? Well, he thought of food twenty-four hours a day. I'm sure he even dreamed about food. He responded to more words describing individual foods—and the descriptive "delicious" that might be applied to some—than one could imagine: kibble, cheese, hamburger, fish, chicken, tomato, carrot, ice cream, cookie, biscuit, and more. Seeing him turn away from a full bowl had not been part of our experience. John and I were very depressed.

One Little Aussie Against the World

The following Wednesday we found ourselves back with Dr. Post for Sparky's second chemotherapy session. Our heads were still spinning from all this. John was trying to be level-headed and practical, but I could see that he wasn't exactly unaffected by the tremendous shift in our lives. I suppose the effects showed more on me; I'm not very good at covering up my feelings. It seemed like life itself had been turned upside down. A few weeks earlier we'd been planning our annual vacation to Vermont. Not far from Bennington is a place with cabins and a large pond, where dogs are allowed. We had gone there for three summers in a row. Sparky loved the place, and we had made several videos of Sparky swimming, Sparky running across open fields doing his "Born Free" imitation, and episodes in restaurants where we whispered to Sparky, who was secretly hidden away under our table in his Sherpa bag. Most likely we had seen our last vacation with Sparky, I thought, but didn't dare say it.

Dr. Post examined Sparky and drew a blood sample. The sample would be sent to the lab and checked for a white-cell count. Chemo tends to lower blood counts, and so the blood must be checked following each treatment. The chemical this time would be Elspar. John bent down to Sparky while the chemical was administered, as he had the week before. "Still...still..."

After a few minutes the procedure ended. We had a lot of questions. In fact, John had typed up a list:

Complimentary treatments?

- ■   *Angiogenesis inhibitors in combination with chemo?*
- ■   *Angiostatin*
- ■   *Endostatin*
- ■   *Thalidomide – has it been tried in treating animals?*
- ■   *Shark's cartilage – ok to try?*
- ■   *Grape seed effective against symptoms?*
- ■   *Any other treatments available and recommended?*
- ■   *Immune system enhancers?*
- ■   *Herbal*
- ■   *Noni juice*
- ■   *General diet – any helpful foods?*

What about holistic veterinarians as an adjunct to traditional treatment?
Do drugs for animals, whether for clinical trials or veterinary treatment, have to be approved by the FDA the same as drugs for humans? How does this work?

General questions

- ■   *How long after surgery before ok to bathe?*
- ■   *Any suggestions for wound (suture) licking?*
- ■   *Diet problems*
- ■   *Withhold food if not eating? Or try another food?*
- ■   *Old diet ok? Cheese ok?*
- ■   *Is some exercise good or is it best to avoid exercise for now?*

John, though not especially a neat or orderly person (you should see his workroom!) can, at times, muster incredible powers of organization. He went down the list with Dr. Post, who patiently addressed each issue—and there were a lot of them! Looking back, I marvel at Dr. Post's patience. He hadn't asked us to write up these reports, yet he never seemed to mind going over each item as if he had all the time in the world—which, believe me, he didn't. If only more of our "people-doctors" could emulate the concern and personal attention so often found in veterinarians! Dr. Post was surprisingly open-minded about experimental drugs and treatments. He okayed the noni juice with a "couldn't hurt" attitude. The tried and tested chemo, however, was to be relied upon first. He didn't scoff at herbal or holistic methods. He recommended a high-fat diet. This, he explained, was because cancer cells are not fed by fat. He suggested a special canned dog food with a high-fat content and said he would give us a prescription for it.

We held our breath for most of the week following Sparky's second chemo—Elspar. John went out and bought a bottle of noni juice, then started giving him a little every day. At first Sparky refused it. You can't blame him; noni tastes something like old prune juice that has turned sour. So John bought a medicine dropper and squeezed the stuff into Sparky's mouth. Sparky's appetite was good, and he was fairly active. Amazingly, during that first week his tumors shrank quite noticeably! That chemo must be powerful stuff, I thought. Sparky's daily menu was revised. We switched over to his new diet, gradually introducing the new and reducing the previous fare. We stocked up on the high-fat canned food. John abandoned the medicine dropper after making the discovery that Sparky didn't mind taking noni straight from his bowl, as long as it was mixed with tomato or fruit juice.

Sparky seemed to be suffering no ill effects from the Elspar. No vomiting or diarrhea. He had received the chemo on a Wednesday, the day on which all his treatments would occur. But on Saturday he seemed to lose his energy. He slept all the time, and barely stood up to eat his meals. On Sunday morning, John put on Sparky's leash for their morning outing. But he was so weak he wouldn't—couldn't—walk.

There is nothing more pathetic than a dog that's too weak to walk. John looked down at him and gave an audible sigh. After a pause, he forced a little cheerfulness: "Okay, Sparky, we *pick-im-up*." He bent down and gently raised the little patient up against his chest. For all six-feet-two of him, my husband looked like a little boy with a beloved teddy bear in his arms.

He took Sparky down the elevator and out to the sidewalk. He set the dog gently down onto the curb, and Sparky, bless him, completed his business in record time. John carried him back to the apartment and lowered Sparky onto the floor. "*Put-im-back*," he said.

Sparky hardly moved the rest of the day. We noticed that he often had panting spells. What did *that* mean?

Then, on Monday, he bounced back remarkably, suddenly regaining full energy! We were overjoyed. "Is this the way it's going to be?" I asked myself. "These emotional highs and lows coming at you at full speed on a daily basis?" And this was just the beginning. I was so delighted to see our little guy scampering around the apartment, but realized we were going to have to get through this one day at a time. He had already begun losing some hair, but we were told to expect this, and were reassured that it would all grow back—though Dr. Post couldn't guarantee that it would be the same color. Sparky's appetite suddenly returned. This roller coaster ride was new to us. Fasten your seat belts, I thought.

For the moment at least, we had our old Sparky back. We realized how much he meant to us. I sat there, watching him wolf down his high-fat dinner one evening and thought back to how things were before we got Sparky.

We had always wanted a dog. I can't say it was a priority though. After we were married, and for several years thereafter, we lived in a fifth-floor walk-up—not exactly ideal for walking a dog two or three times a day. In those days, John was the musical director for the Fanfare Theatre Ensemble—a children's theater company whose repertory included many shows for which he had written the music. He often went on tour with the company, and would be on the road for weeks at a time. This continued after 1976, when we moved into the high-rise where we are now.

Sometimes in the summer he'd do stock theater, also as musical director. If I didn't accompany him I would invariably visit for a few weeks, depending on where the theater was located. If it were near the ocean or a resort, that would be our vacation. We spent many summers this way.

Between John's frequent travels out of town and my working in an office four days a week it was, again, not exactly an ideal situation for having a dog. Then there was the sticky matter of our lease in the high-rise, which strictly prohibited tenants from owning dogs. It was a brand new building, and the agents who rented the apartments were very cavalier about the "no dogs" clause. We told the rental agent that we didn't have a dog now, but asked if it would it be okay if we got one later. He told us that it would be okay and not to worry; the clause wouldn't be enforced. However, tenants who didn't like neighbors keeping dogs in the building were told just the opposite! Many would-be tenants signed the lease and brought their animals with them. Barely had they settled into their new digs when the management, acting on complaints by this anti-dog crowd, threatened the dog owners with eviction unless they got rid of their canines. A few gave their pets to family members who lived elsewhere. The others left the building rather than give up their dogs.

Now that we have Sparky I can certainly understand that. I could sort of see it at the time, too, but not to the extent I do now. Dennis Prager used to have a talk show on the radio in New York. He is still on the air in Los Angeles, I believe. I remember him discussing a tricky question: "If your dog and a stranger were drowning and you could only save one, which of the two would you rescue?" He was appalled, he said—and I with him—that so many people said they would save their dog. Today I'm not so sure. In any event I can't swim, so I couldn't help either one. How's that for a cop-out!

As time passed, though, our neighbors in the building started sneaking in dogs, mostly little ones that could be taken out in shoulder bags. I know one woman who confessed she had never been without a Chihuahua.

But, little by little, the no-dogs situation changed. This was due, basically, to a revision in the city's statutes. The new laws stipulated that if a tenant "openly and notoriously harbored a dog" for three months and the landlord took no action against him, he could keep the dog no matter what the lease said. The landlords, however, often took action before the end of the three-month period and sued the tenants. The irony was that the judges very often came down on the side of the tenants anyway.

Should we go ahead and get a dog? we wondered. We had always wanted one, and by then John was teaching; touring became a thing of the past and I was working only two days a week. Would we be able to *harbor* one, *openly* and *notoriously*, for three months without being thrown out of our home? There was no guarantee we would succeed. How would we get him in and out of the building? There was an entrance through the subterranean parking garage. Could we sneak him in and out that way—openly and notoriously?

We decided to risk it.

We wanted to do things right and set out to do some research. What kind of dog would be happy in a city apartment? Which breed? What size? Even though we both had had dogs as kids, we realized we didn't know much about these creatures.

The first book we bought was an illustrated *Handbook of Dogs*, edited by Roger Caras. It had a clear, beautiful color photograph of every breed recognized by the American Kennel

Club up until 1985, the year the book was published. The book proved invaluable. We had great fun looking at the pictures and reading the accompanying descriptions. Every breed had something to recommend it, though the larger ones were obviously not suited to our situation. We kept going back to picture number thirty-one, the Australian terrier. Neither John nor I had ever heard of the breed, much less seen one. For years we'd enjoyed watching the Westminster Show, televised from Madison Square Garden, but we couldn't recall ever having seen an Australian terrier there. Even so, this alert little terrier struck us as perfect. Every feature of this dog as characterized in the book described an animal that struck us both as ideal for our needs and preferences. It seemed like a good apartment dog, conveniently small but still a real dog. They were easy to get along with, needed little grooming, and had few if any notable health problems. The more we read the more we liked.

But where to find one? As it happened, it was January, and the Westminster Show was only a few weeks away. John had discovered that one could purchase tickets to the Best of Breed competitions at the Garden. These contests were not televised but were open to the public. After finding out exactly when the Australian terrier trials were scheduled, we excitedly got ourselves down to Madison Square Garden.

The Westminster is what's known as a "benching" show, which means that besides viewing the proceedings from a seat in the stands, visitors can go "backstage" (under the Garden's seating tiers) and see all the contestants, who are assigned to specific locations by breed. This vast, curved space was filled to capacity with every breed of canine—large, small, and in between. Some wanted to make sure their presence was being noticed. Others were being groomed; a few were asleep. Their owners were with them.

I had never seen so many dogs in one place! Most all were crated, but some smaller breeds were in squared-off pens filled with wood shavings. I particularly remember three or four Affenpinschers penned in this way who were too cute for words. There were several Australian terriers and we were really taken with their looks and behavior. Their breeders or owners seemed very happy with their charges but, unfortunately, had none for sale. They did give us the names of several breeders, though. The owner of two entrants was also a breeder, but she had no puppies due in the near future. It turned out she was also the president of the Australian Terrier Association. She promised to send us a printed list of all AKC breeders in the country. One lady from Wisconsin told us of a breeder in Michigan whom she knew had Aussies for sale. But Michigan wasn't exactly next door.

Soon it was time to go back to the main arena for the Australian terrier Best of Breed competition. There must have been six or eight Best of Breed contests occurring at the same time on the huge subdivided floor (which on another occasion might host a basketball game or the circus). John and I circled around and found a couple of seats by the Aussies. John counted sixteen of them. They looked a lively lot; it was impossible to pick a favorite. One kept jumping in the air for the entertainment of a fellow contestant. Another was stretched out flat on his belly with his hind legs extending straight out to the rear in what John would later call the "tadpole" position.

"Look!" John said. "Have you every seen dogs lie like that?"

Then another one followed suit, lounging in this position amid the circus-like frolicking of the other Aussies. It was the most charming thing I ever saw.

I can't say which of the ten or eleven entrants was selected. They all looked irresistible to us. Our minds were made up: we would get an Aussie.

This, it turned out, was easier said than done. In no time at all we exhausted the list of contacts we had gotten at the Garden. Even the list of breeders from the Australian Terrier Association proved no more successful in terms of providing us with a puppy. "Call back in June," or some other future date seemed to be the universal response. Where we once had summarily rejected the idea of venturing as far as Michigan, we changed our mind and called Mary Jo, the breeder in Ann Arbor. She had several puppies, she informed us, a male and a female of about six months, and three or four much younger puppies. She was prepared to sell the older ones, she said, but she didn't know about the little ones yet. Breeders, of course, want to know if a puppy has show dog potential. This is not discernible until a puppy has developed sufficiently. Aussies are uniformly black at birth, with floppy ears that don't perk until later. Sometimes the ears never perk, or other imperfections show up that disqualify a puppy as a show dog. And show dogs were Mary Jo's first priority.

At one point she asked why I wanted a dog. I mumbled something about always having wanted a dog because, "I'd like to walk around with it." This sentence remains stuck in my mind because this, surely, had to be one of the worst answers to the question. John must've done better because she seemed satisfied. The price would be $400 to $450 cash.

Most people would have had the dog shipped by air. We decided to drive to Ann Arbor and back. John's midterm break was coming up, and he would have more than a week off. We would rent a car (like many New Yorkers, owning a car was just too much of a hassle for us) and travel via Pittsburgh, where John had been born, and where his alma mater is located. I had never been to Pittsburgh, and he couldn't wait to show me Carnegie Mellon, known as Carnegie Tech in his day. We would stay overnight and continue on to Michigan the next day.

On February 20, 1995, we left New York in our rental car. It was a cold, cloudless day—excellent driving weather. But by the time we neared Pittsburgh that afternoon, the sky was turning that particular gray that foretells snow in the offing. I hadn't realized how picturesquely Pittsburgh was situated. After years of hearing Pittsburgh jokes on late-night TV, I had braced myself for steel mills and factories belching out filthy smoke and soot. But I was struck by the city's natural beauty, which not even the murky winter sky could hide.

We toured the Carnegie campus, and John took me through the Fine Arts building with its many rooms and sky-lit art studios familiar to him from his student days. Some were exactly as he remembered them. So, while the trip was marked by the excitement and anticipation over the prospect of acquiring a dog, it was also nostalgic for him. We visited the house built by his father—long deceased—and now occupied by strangers. We saw the church where his mother had married his stepfather—both also now gone. He showed me the red-brick school building he had walked to every day as a child growing up during World War II, still in operation and essentially unchanged in appearance. All in all, it was an emotional day, the distant past mingling with the future shock of a new family member.

All that comes to mind when I think of our ride from Pittsburgh through Ohio to Ann Arbor are the icy roads. Miles and miles of treacherous highway and weather reports on the car radio promising more of the same up ahead. Bleak vistas and snow-covered fields. All the way. Just before the Michigan border we spotted a mileage sign that included "Ann Arbor." We both gave a little cheer and then promptly got lost.

John had carefully mapped out our route, but this was before detailed Internet route-maps. John backtracked and got us on the right road again. Making one wrong turn, one might end up in California, I thought. Then, as we crossed the border into the state of Michigan, the sun appeared and the snow stopped! Blinding, sunny white landscape! Clear blue sky! A good sign.

We found the motel where we had reserved a room and immediately called Mary Jo, who gave us driving directions to her house. Excited, we drove there immediately, without even freshening up from the car trip or even grabbing a bite to eat. When we knocked on the front door, a voice from inside told us to go around to the back. In the yard behind the gate were a dozen or so small dogs, all fiercely barking a welcome. There had been a recent thaw in the area, and what no doubt had been a snow-covered back yard was now pretty much mud. But the dogs didn't mind the mud or the cold. This is the picture I imagine next to the word *enthusiasm* in the dictionary: these ebullient little terriers, all yapping and yelping and springing in the air and at each other for the sheer joy of it. I couldn't stop laughing. Mary Jo came out and opened the gate for us to enter the yard. The dogs followed us inside to the kitchen, their enthusiasm never flagging.

There was no place to sit. Mary Jo brought in a chair for me from some other room. Scrambling over each other in a sort of crib were the baby Aussies, only slightly larger than hamsters, their as-yet undocked tails wagging at our approach. In a corner were three black miniature poodles, very much the grownups in this boisterous menagerie. Cats, their tails up in the air, marched among the canines as though they weren't there. The poodles, knowing full well that every time strangers arrived they would walk off with a dog, came to sit near us. "Take one of us!" they seemed to say. "We are so much more civilized than those wild terriers." And so they were indeed.

It proved impossible to select one of the Aussies, since they would not sit still. We couldn't even identify the ones Mary Jo was prepared to sell—her own personal dogs were mixed in—because of the constant play. I tried to pull one onto my lap, but he would have none of it.

I couldn't begin to make a choice, even if I eliminated the babies from the selection pool. I felt as I had watching the Best of Breed in Madison Square Garden; they all struck me as irresistible.

I turned to John. "You make the choice. I can't."

"Okay, I'll try."

Mary Jo tried to make it easier. "Come on, everybody!" she shouted to the dogs, and chased them all into the yard, where they soon exhausted themselves and came to sit on the steps outside the glass storm door.

One puppy caught John's attention. "What's that one's name?" he asked.

"He doesn't have a name yet."

The puppy was moving away from the door where they stood, but stopped, turned slightly, cocked his head and stared John squarely in the eye. That was it for John. The deal was sealed. This would become our dog, and we would have to come up with an appropriate name for him. He was born on the Fourth of July, 1994, and was now seven months old. Mary Jo told us that his mama's name was Can-Do and his papa's was Jumpin' Jack Flash. His sister (sold) had been dubbed "Rocket."

Mary Jo—earlier, on the telephone—had insisted that we buy a crate for our new puppy. When John, in a subsequent call, quoted her the price of a crate in New York, she assured him he could buy one at half that price in Ann Arbor. She now reminded us we had to buy this item.

"Plus a leash," she added. "Then you'll need to get some food. They have everything you'll need down at PetsMart. Toys and whatever." She also instructed us about the ride home.

"Don't make an overnight layover," she insisted. " Drive straight through in one stretch."

This sounded like a reasonable request. It would be traumatic enough for the doggie to suddenly lose all his frolicking playmates and be stuck with two strangers.

As for the crate, we weren't too sure about it, though Mary Jo seemed a great believer in crates. Later, when the dogs were all back in the house, we got a glimpse of another room through the kitchen door. There was crate upon crate, each with its doggie owner lying possessively in front of it. Anyway, we would need something to transport him, so, after John paid her, we decided to buy the crate and whatever else was needed.

But first our new family member was to be checked out by a vet. Although Mary Jo was a veterinarian herself she wanted the puppy to receive a clean bill of health from an independent source. This was not a bad idea, we thought.

We made the short trip to the vet's office, John driving our rental car, following Mary Jo's station wagon with our doggie inside. There our Aussie was placed on the examining table by an orderly, who promptly mistook him for a stray! This certainly pointed up how dirty he was, running in that muddy yard day in and day out. I resolved to give him a bath first thing when we got home. He didn't protest being manhandled by the vet—didn't snap or bite—and stood quite patiently and resignedly through the process. The vet pronounced him fit and hale, but shy. And stubborn, I thought. He refused to set one paw on the highly polished tiles of one section of the office floor. Steps he flew up without hesitation, but this slippery surface made him recoil. He dug in his paws and wouldn't budge. "They're very conscious of surfaces," offered Mary Jo.

Judging by his cautious behavior at the veterinarian's, we realized this little creature had never known anything other than Mary Jo's house and yard and his gamboling playmates. He was seven months old and conditioned to his surroundings. And, needless to say, very happy to go back there. After depositing the dog back at Mary Jo's place, she joined John and me in our car and we set out for PetsMart, where we bought a crate, two huge sacks of kibble, toys, and a few dozen other things besides.

We piled up our purchases in the trunk, then Mary Jo gave John directions to a bookstore where she insisted we buy a book called *The Art of Raising a Puppy*. She also wanted us to buy something called *Civilized City Canines*, which was written by a friend of hers, but the store didn't have it. John invited Mary Jo to have dinner with us—we were starved—and she accepted.

I recall nothing of the restaurant or my meal except that it was awful (John claimed it was my fault for ordering fish in a landlocked place) and that Mary Jo only drank water. No beer or wine for her; "*No*-sir!" she cried to the waiter. She's been around dogs too long, I thought.

After dropping off Mary Jo, we returned to the motel, trying to come up with a name. At one point John suggested "Sparky" and that name struck me as just about perfect. He was born on the Fourth of July, after all. And, to be sure, he sparkled, springing and tearing through that back yard. Mary Jo, too, declared it perfect when we went to pick up our Sparky early the next day. Sparky himself was completely indifferent to his perfect name, no matter how often we addressed him by it.

Before we headed back, Mary Jo reminded us that he needed to be neutered as soon as possible after our return home, or else she wouldn't send us the registration papers. When breeders sell a dog that's not breeding quality, they want to make sure that he's not bred. Sparky's front paws turned out somewhat, and this was considered sufficient reason to disqualify him from mating. We readily promised, since it had been impressed upon us from many sides—not just Mary Jo— that neutering was in the best interest of the dog. She gave us a form for the vet to sign, certifying the neutering had been done, and instructed us to mail it back.

We thanked Mary Jo and said goodbye. With Sparky in his crate on the back seat, we started on the long way back. Mary Jo had given us a T-shirt so that Sparky would have a familiar scent in his crate, to minimize the trauma of being snatched by two strangers from the only home he had ever known.

Ann Arbor disappeared behind us. Our little rental car zoomed toward New York City. Sparky would never again see his playmates, Mary Jo, or those reassuring, familiar surround- ings. He was headed for a completely new life. And, though we didn't realize it at the time, so were we.

The Joy of Anticipation

The twelve-hour journey back to Manhattan seemed more like twelve days, even though the roads were clear and the traffic was light. We had our dog, but we couldn't wait to get him home and out of that crate. We stopped only to pick up something to eat or to let Sparky take a tinkle or a drink of water. Every time the car slowed down for whatever reason he would stand up in the crate, then settle down again as it regained speed. He seemed very docile and a bit frightened when John put on the leash and took him for a little walk.

As happy as we were to finally reach New York late that evening, John and I were both anxious about how to get our new addition to the family inside our apartment building without being seen. Some of our neighbors were very anti-dog and would have done anything to keep the building dog-free. Others were indifferent. The majority, though, I'd venture to guess, liked dogs even if they didn't have one. It was the first type, needless to say, we had to avoid at all costs.

John had devised a plan. The underground garage, though part of our building, was run independently. We would park there and give the attendant twenty bucks. This would buy us enough time to conceal our tell-tale pet store purchases, not to mention our pet and crate, and take the elevator straight up to the 27th floor without having to parade everything through the lobby. The parking attendant was a dour individual, but cash mollified him.

All went as planned. We unloaded the car, and John piled everything into the elevator while I held the door. He put the crate at the very rear of the car, hiding it as best he could with our suitcases and garment bags. Even so, we were nervous wrecks by the time the elevator moved and—oh no!—stopped at the lobby. It was long past the hour when people came home from work. We had hoped the elevator would bypass the ground floor, but in such a large building this proved a silly notion. Two people got on. John and I huddled in front of the crate, resting our many shopping bags atop the pile. Sparky thus far had cooperated beautifully, not making a peep during the entire procedure. But would it last? What if he started to yap or make a fuss suddenly? The people, luckily, got off before we reached our floor.

At long last we were back in our apartment, crate and dog safely inside. John opened the crate door and let Sparky have a look at his new home. He was not impressed. He came out and promptly lifted his leg against the coffee table. "No!" I cried, and he stopped.

Mary Jo had assured us that Sparky was housebroken. Not only that, but he had been to obedience class, she said. If this was true, and we had no reason to doubt it, it had left no impression on Sparky. He did seem to understand the word "no," though.

While John returned to the garage to remove the car before the attendant's mollified state expired, I tried to coax

Sparky onto our balcony. Nothing doing. Just as he had refused to put one paw on the slippery waxed floor in the vet's office, he now stubbornly refused to set one foot out of the balcony door. He dug in his paws and that was that. John returned and set up the crate beside our bed. We put Sparky in it for the night. In spite of all the tensions of the day, we had no trouble sleeping, and didn't hear a peep out of Sparky.

The next day the difficulties continued. We'd imagined ourselves well-prepared. We'd done research. Read books. We were responsible individuals, John and I. We followed the instructions in the books to the letter, but our puppy didn't behave as prescribed. That morning we immediately cordoned off a section of our hallway with adjustable wooden barriers—child gates actually—and covered the carpet with heavy plastic. The puppy's space was supposed to be made gradually bigger as he adjusted to his new surroundings and learned "to go" on paper.

Sparky ignored the paper and tried to jump over the barrier. When he didn't make it the first time, he sprang up onto his crate—which was placed close to the barrier—and jumped over from there.

"The little devil!" I cried.

"We'll have to move the crate further back," said John, "away from the gate."

John slid the crate back, a good distance from the barrier. Sparky again jumped up onto the roof of the crate. He looked at the top edge of the barrier in preparation to jump over it. But he hesitated, calculating that the distance was too great—he'd never make it.

He jumped back to the floor. After a pause he sauntered back to the wall, away from the crate and the gate. Suddenly, he turned, took off running and leapt up and over the crate, not landing on it but merely using it to get an extra push with his hind legs as he went sailing over the barrier into the living room. He looked at us as if to say "Wasn't that great?"

John was amazed. "Up until now I was never aware that animals understood the scientific principles of momentum." He shook his head. "Wow..."

The gates were adjustable in width, allowing them to be wedged tightly into a doorway or across a narrow hall. John raised the gate in order to make it higher. No problem. Sparky simply flattened himself and wriggled out underneath.

While we were amused by his resourcefulness and admired his indomitable spirit, it became clear that steps would have to be taken to housebreak this dog. He went where he pleased—within the confines of his space to be sure—but never where he was *supposed* to go. The bathroom, to which he had access, and the paper there remained untouched. *Something* would have to be done *soon*, but what?

Taking him out was also a problem. And not just because we had to hide him. Poor Sparky, accustomed to the quiet of his heretofore suburban digs, was terrified of New York City. The noise, the traffic, the constant bustle petrified him. When an ambulance passed, siren blaring, Sparky would run for the nearest door and scratch on it desperately, trying to find indoor cover. The first time John took him out, a day after our return from Ann Arbor, the dog became so unhinged he befouled himself—unnoticed at first. Then upon his return home shook

himself, setting the you-know-what flying all over the foyer.
Well, we *wanted* a dog and we *had* one!

Now, here we were, years later. Lymphoma.
Chemotherapy. How unpredictable the future is! I watched
Sparky finish his high-fat meal. Then he looked at me: "Got
more?" he was asking. I couldn't help smiling. "What a little
trooper you are," I told him.

The week following Sparky's second chemotherapy
treatment certainly hadn't been as good as the previous week.
While his most recent injection had been Elspar, it's difficult to
say if that drug alone was responsible—weeks can pass before
side effects show up. For the moment, though, he seemed
trouble-free.

On Wednesday morning John saw those little tell-tale
white "rice" things in Sparky's stool. "He's got a tapeworm
again," he announced. This meant a trip over to Animal
General for the magic tapeworm pill. Sparky had had a
tapeworm twice in the past, and I remember how alarmed John
and I would become. Now, of course, a tapeworm seemed a
minor concern.

That evening found us back with Dr. Post for more
chemo. Yet another chemical this time—Cytoxan.

We told Dr. Post about the roller-coaster week we had
just experienced, and John produced his written questions:

*How many different specific **types** of chemotherapy treat-*
ments can we anticipate?

What is the biggest contributing factor to his excessive thirst (disease, Prednisone, chemotherapy treatments)?

Could his ravenous appetite have been partly due to the tapeworm? Or, is his appetite related principally to the cancer or treatments?

Sparky is six. When first diagnosed, an intern (at Animal Medical Center) suggested that his age fell within the typical profile for lymphoma. True?

What is the possibility of Sparky receiving experimental treatment? Any clinical trials?

How did Sparky's white blood cell count hold up this past week, as compared to the first week of therapy?

Dr. Post went through the questions, answering each in turn. There would be four chemicals in rotation. After a certain period, he would drop two from the cycle and add another. Sparky's thirst and panting spells came from the treatment, mainly the Prednisone pills. His appetite was also due to the Prednisone. Many dogs contract lymphoma at age five and six; this is typical. As for clinical trials, Dr. Post was open to the idea but suggested that he would only consider this option if the chemotherapy didn't keep Sparky in remission. The white blood cell count was good.

Sparky received his Cytoxan injection. We left Animal General. "Well, what fate awaits the three of us *this* week?" John asked. My thoughts exactly.

On September 6, 2000, the doctor introduced another chemical into the cycle of therapeutic poisons he would administer. Our new vocabulary word for this visit to Dr. Post was "Adriamycin." Upon first hearing the word, I thought that it wouldn't be long before John was at his computer looking it up on the Internet.

By now, Sparky was in remission from the cancer. The chemo was definitely doing its thing. We entered the tiny examination room with Sparky in John's arms, ready for the chemo treatment. The reason John carried Sparky from the waiting room to the exam room was not because Sparky was weak, it was because Sparky was exceptionally afraid of having his nails cut. Just past the row of exam rooms was the door to the dreaded operating room, where Sparky's paws had often been assaulted by clipper-wielding nurses and orderlies. With him, it was not simply a matter of "I'd rather not go through this right now." It was "get me out of here" time. He was so terrified of this procedure that he regularly pooped on the perpetrators of the horror. The receivers of this indignity were surprisingly good-natured about it.

"Well, how's he doing?" Dr. Post asked.

"Great," John answered, and handed Dr. Post a written report. We waited in silence as the doctor scanned the document. Sparky's third week had been the best so far. The Cytoxan seemed to agree with him; at least it caused no major problems. We had come to understand that bad reactions to the chemotherapy did not necessarily occur immediately after the administration of the drug. Often the side-effect, whatever it might be, would turn up on the third or fourth day after treatment.

The first day after the Cytoxan had been good. We then waited for the "bad" day, but none came. Sparky's energy level remained at 100 percent the entire week. His appetite had been excellent; there were no incidents of vomiting or diarrhea. His panting spells had stopped. This was most likely due to the fact that the Prednisone dosage had been cut in half. A hint of a smile crept across Dr. Post's face as he read further:

> *...He seemed to crave more exercise, and took us for longer walks, and even tore around Central Park yesterday. Surprisingly to us, his water intake went back to normal levels, and there were no indoor "accidents"...*

The week had gone well—but our main worry was keeping our dog in remission. This was how it would be—if Sparky had problems we'd worry that he was going out of remission. If he did well, we'd worry about how long the good spell would last before he might go out of remission. Seeing those tumors shrink down to nothing, watching him romp in the park, enjoying the sight of his wolfing down his dinner again—all these things were a joy to behold, but it was a joy that competed with a lump in my throat. The positive things spawned hope, but the hope stirred feelings that perhaps we were expecting too much, that we were tempting fate by daring to exhibit optimism.

I told myself that, no matter what, I would keep a positive attitude. John's more of a natural worrier than I, but he also tried to keep on the bright side. "Worrying won't help," he'd say.

At the end of John's report, the doctor came to the inevitable questions. The first question dealt with the possibility of additional treatment to compliment the chemotherapy.

Dr. Post read the last part aloud. "Would Sparky benefit from seeing a veterinarian who practices alternative medicine? Any recommendations?" Looking up from his paper, he said, "Sure. There's only one veterinarian I would recommend for this." He wrote the doctor's name and phone number on a slip of paper and handed it to John. "He's in Westchester. You can give him a call."

Dr. Post, while being self-assured and confident of his own methods, was wonderfully open-minded about other treatments, new drugs and techniques, and what was going on in his field outside his own experience. His willingness to consider innovation and experimentation was all the encouragement John needed to become actively involved in seeking out new information on different treatments and clinical trials. The part of John's report indicating that we were giving Sparky regular doses of noni juice and fish oil was accepted without remark or objection. John had read about fish oil on the Internet. Apparently there were studies to show that it boosted survival times. Most of these studies were conducted using human data, but human diseases bear a definite, if not exact, resemblance to canines. So we mixed a few drops into his meals—we didn't want to miss out on *anything* that might help.

The last question on John's list referred to the blood sample taken the previous week. How had Sparky's white blood cell count held up?

"White cells are fine." This ended the written portion of our visit. Dr. Post crumpled up the paper and dropped it into the waste bin.

The rest of the visit followed the routine of the last one: stethoscope exam, temperature taken with rectal thermometer, checking Sparky's entire body with the hands, and the chemo injection.

Sure enough, as soon as we got home, John was on the computer searching for the low-down on Adriamycin.

The generic name of Adriamycin is Doxorubicin. The category of the drug is listed as "antineoplastic," another nice five-dollar medical word. John's search for the definition of the word turned up some interesting information on "antineoplaston therapy." It turned out that antineoplastons are not like other chemotherapy drugs, which typically are intended to kill cancer cells *and* healthy cells. Apparently what antineoplastons do is to interrupt the activity of the "ras oncogene." Hmm. Reading further, we found out that this meant it stopped the cancer cell's ability to divide endlessly. Sounded good.

What about the side effects of Adriamycin? The printout included an endless list, but nothing that was too serious. This drug looked perhaps promising in that respect. Did we dare hope the next week would be another good one?

Life—A Long Rehearsal for a Short Performance

Each time Sparky received his chemotherapy treatment, I was struck by the courage he exhibited. He obviously did *not* like being held down on that stainless steel table with a needle stuck in his leg, yet he hardly ever struggled or fidgeted during this unnatural procedure. He just lay there, looking into John's face with those soulful eyes, seeming to accept it all, placing his trust, if not in the doctor, in his owners and their assurance that no harm would befall him.

He had not always been this trusting and intrepid. I thought back to when he was a puppy, seemingly afraid of the world itself, at least as far as New York City was concerned...

Sal, a colleague of John's who lived a block away, had a pug that he took to the park nearly every afternoon. John was then teaching at the Cultural Arts Center, a high school for artistically inclined kids in Syosset, Long Island. On their drives to work, which took an hour-plus each way, they had plenty of opportunities to chat. Sal knew all about Sparky's antics and fears and the trouble we had housebreaking him.

Brandy, the little pug, could have been the poster dog for paper training, she was so good at it. She also was completely at ease with the sounds of New York City streets. Sal suggested that John and Sparky go along with them to Riverside Park one afternoon. Sparky, being so dog-oriented, was sure to follow Brandy. And so he did.

Sparky forgot about screeching tires, buses, and other mammoth vehicles. He concentrated solely on Brandy, and his attention flagged only when confronted with the half-dozen or so other dogs in the park's dog run. Brandy was a "people dog" with a minimal, if any, interest in canine goings-on. She barely acknowledged Sparky's existence. But Sparky was immediately at home in the dog run, going so far as to lunge at a Bernese mountain dog, who luckily for Sparky was a good sport about it.

After this introductory exposure to Riverside Park, our dog was forever poised to return there. Once outside the door, he would run, docked tail in the air, as if his life depended on it, and head straight for the park that ran along the Hudson River. Coming back from the park, however, was like dragging home a sack of potatoes. Many times I was forced to hold a liver treat in front of his nose to get him to move. "The dog from hell," as I described him to John at those times.

We had met a lady there with a corgi named Baxter who became one of Sparky's early pals. This lady complained of a problem identical to our own, regarding paper training. "I've given it up. It doesn't work," she said. "At least not with Baxter. I'm taking him out several times a day now. It's a lot of bother, but it works."

Another dog owner had told John of an obedience class his Boston terrier attended and how the dog's behavior had improved after that. This sounded like a good idea for *our* dog!

Sparky was very wild. To take him for a walk wasn't the pleasant, relaxing experience I had envisioned when I had foolishly said to Mary Jo, "I'd like to walk around with it." He would pull at his leash, veer this way and that, poke in the gutter, then suddenly fly into a doorway at some unexpected noise. One of the books warned about Aussies being "lightning quick." With this in mind, I would hold Sparky's leash with both hands but, even so, he had already escaped my grip twice: once, in the park when I despaired of finding him until a man pointed him out high up on an embankment; another time in front of our building where a girl—bless her—chased after him and stepped on his leash before he could dash into the traffic on Amsterdam Avenue.

For all his running for cover into doorways, he refused to enter shops, the post office, or the bank. Once forced inside the bank, say, or the camera shop, I had to watch him constantly. The word "No!" was always on the tip of my tongue since the first gesture he was inclined to make was lifting a leg. He was better with John, but not much.

We were still entering and exiting our building through the basement parking garage in order to avoid the eyes of our security guards, who sat at a desk in the main lobby. The guards were usually friendly enough, but we couldn't be sure they wouldn't inform the management about Sparky. The parking garage people, we figured, couldn't care less, since they didn't work for the building. Sparky didn't mind zigzagging through the parked cars on his way out. There is a long drainage grate that stretches across the floor of the entrance to the garage, where the vehicles go in and out. The openings in the grate are about an inch wide, too large for Sparky to negotiate without his legs going through. He quickly learned to make a nice neat jump over the grate. John started saying "Jump!" just as Sparky went over, and he quickly learned that word and what it meant. He'll still jump on command.

Meanwhile, we had taken Sparky to Westside Veterinary Center (the closer Animal General didn't exist then) to see about having him neutered and had received an appointment for surgery on March 13. We decided not to wait, though, for this event to enroll him in obedience school. John had heard that "Follow My Lead" was a good one, and made arrangements for classes. We also decided to follow Baxter's mistress's example and give up on the paper-training business.

In order to reach Cultural Arts by 8:00 A.M., John had to leave home around 6:00. He took Sparky for his first outing before his departure. Then at 11:00 or so I'd take him to the park for a short spell. Upon his return in the afternoon, John again would take him to the park, and then once more, late at night for a utility "quickie." As Baxter's owner said, "It's a lot of bother, but it works." It proved a wise decision, as did the decision to enroll Sparky in obedience training.

The classes—there would be eight of them—were held weekly in a church basement gymnasium. As the weather grew warmer, they were transferred to various outdoor locales. I went along with John the first time to see what it was all about.

Sparky liked the place right off. So many dogs! How could he not? He also, surprisingly, was on his best behavior, except when a Westie called Oba was near, in which case he danced a little jig.

Sparky has always approached dogs entirely differently than people. With dogs he is outgoing, and with some particular dogs—we never know just why these certain ones—he is simply effervescent. At first, he'll look at his potential playmate and spring up on his hind legs, making a paddling motion with his forepaws. The object of this attention typically does a double-take. Then Sparky will jump straight up, all fours off the ground, do a 360-degree spin in mid-air, and land nose to nose with the other dog. Large or small, he is comfortable with all sorts of canines—Rotweillers, Chihuahuas, you name it. Not that he isn't discriminating. A few dogs—again, who knows why?—are simply not his type. John often says, "What a character," and I have to agree. Sparky is something else.

The other dog owners attending the training sessions couldn't help but single out Sparky. First of all, there's his famous gait. Sparky doesn't just walk, he prances like a pony, as if he owns the place. Even though the shortest people tower above little Sparky, he makes them feel he's looking down at them as he bobs along, pony-like, with an intelligence likely to come across as arrogance. John told me about a doorman who observed, as he and Sparky passed by his building, "That dog walks like a *king*!" And so he does.

The owners in class, expecting typical doggie behavior, were disappointed when Sparky didn't instantly wag his tail and slobber over them with puppyish affection. He looks so cute that people generally expect this type of greeting but, unless you're an old pal, it doesn't happen.

A week into classes, Sparky was neutered. I took him to Westside Veterinary Center in the morning, since John had to work. John and I had mixed feelings about this process. It seemed the best thing to do—there are so many unwanted dogs in this world—but, still, it is a mutilation. We humans perform so many alterations on dogs' bodies: we dock their tails or operate on their ears just because we like the way it looks. We create breeds that have built-in problems, such as respiratory troubles (*i.e.* pugs), hip displasia ailments (collies and other large dogs), skin problems (bichons). Still, all things considered, neutering seems the kindest thing in the long run, preventing unwanted little ones that might only be destroyed. And it does *not* change their behavior—not if Sparky is any indication.

We went to pick up Sparky the following afternoon, happy that the surgery had gone well. But if we had hoped Sparky would wag his tail upon seeing us we were disappointed.

At this point, four weeks after his arrival, Sparky still did not respond to his name or wag his tail at us. Only dogs— Baxter, Oba, another Brandy, a "generic" dog who wasn't much in the looks department but whom Sparky loved—could induce him to wag his tail. Our dog's taste was his own, not ours. And this Brandy, twice as big as Sparky, loved him back.

The classes, however, were a turning point in Sparky's demeanor. He bonded with John and took the commands to heart. The "drop-it" command alone was worth the price of admission: $225 for the eight lessons. Out of the three female instructors, Sparky liked Phyllis best.

But Sparky, being Sparky, had to be willful. He got it into his head that only John should take him out. If I attempted to take him, he would dig in his paws and not budge. If John was at home he would have to stop playing the piano, correcting papers, or whatever he was doing, and take Sparky's leash from me to guide him out the door. Once in the hall, the leash was transferred back into my hands. Sparky would then willingly follow me even though John had gone back inside. Go figure. This routine went on longer than I care to remember. However, when John wasn't home, Sparky happily trotted out with me, though never quite as happily as with John.

Finally, during obedience training, we were able to take down the barriers and get rid of the plastic carpet covers. We gave Sparky the run of the place, one room at a time, and with either John or me in it. In the living room, Sparky promptly ran into the glass balcony door, which gave him—and his cute little nose— quite a shock. Soon afterward, he saw himself in our floor-length mirror and barked loudly at this perceived intruder. This must have been the first time he barked—at home I mean. If it weren't for his frantic vocal reactions to little kids we might have concluded he couldn't bark at all, for he was completely quiet indoors. For anyone wanting to "harbor" a dog (never mind "openly and notoriously") Sparky certainly was the ideal candidate.

John put flower-shaped stickers on the balcony door glass, but Sparky had already identified the problem, just as he had with his refection in the mirror. It was anybody's guess what he thought of the creature barking at him in the mirror, but he decided to treat it as he did the images on TV. If there was no scent and the image didn't materialize it was not worthy of his attention.

Sparky enjoyed his new freedom and seemed to reward us for it by being especially good. It is said that terriers are very clean, and our little terrier tried to do his category proud. I'm not saying there wasn't the occasional accident, but he did his best to please. Not only that, but outside on the sidewalks he always made for the curb to do his business. We had never taught him that.

Was it instinct? Or had someone trained him? Had our Aussie been owned by someone before us? Had he been called by another name given by a previous owner? Was that why at seven months old he was still at the breeder's? Was that the reason he didn't respond to his perfect name? Mary Jo had told us he was housebroken and had attended obedience class. Do breeders housebreak puppies? Do they send them for obedience training? Except for the teeny ones, Mary Jo had given names to all the other puppies, some younger than Sparky. At seven months, Sparky alone had remained nameless.

We never got the answers to these questions. In fact, it was a long time before John and I even thought to ask these questions. Because for all our prep work and thinking ourselves well-informed, we, in reality, weren't very know-ledgeable about dogs.

For instance, the crate. Sparky liked his crate. So much so, in fact, we were prepared to support Mary Jo in her belief in crates. After he had tried out corners and nooks in the living room, Sparky would invariably return to settle in his crate. He'd jump into the armchair or hop up onto the couch—our brand new green leather couch on which we had vowed not to let him place a paw. And, after treating John or me to a momentary snuggle there, he would hurry back to his crate. At night John would move the crate into the bedroom. And once or twice, when he'd placed him on the bed, Sparky, after a short stay, would jump off to go sleep in his crate. He didn't even mind being locked inside it, so long as he could see what went on outside.

The windows in our apartment have removable panes and, once the weather allowed, we took them to the balcony to give them a thorough cleansing and hosing down. Sparky, being such an enthusiastic jumper and unfamiliar with the procedure, couldn't be trusted on the loose with no windows in place. He liked to investigate everything, so John locked Sparky in the crate and placed it where he could follow the action. Sparky seemed perfectly content.

But we began to suspect that he was not happy locked in there when we were not home. Whenever we went out, for however short a time, we'd find the carpet that lay on the bottom of his crate chewed to shreds. Ironically, it was this frenetic chewing that convinced us not to leave the crate open. God knows what havoc he might wreak if given full rein of the apartment during our absence!

But we obviously couldn't always be home with him. The next time we prepared to go out, John set up the cassette recorder and switched it on as we left. What we heard when we played the tape upon our return upset us no end. Our poor little puppy had cried pitifully the entire time we were gone. We assumed it was the entire time because we hadn't the heart to play the tape through to the end. I threw the cassette in the trash together with the tattered piece of carpet while John dismantled the crate. The door was removed once and for all, and the two plastic halves of the crate itself, top and bottom, were separated. He inverted the top part and nested it into the bottom piece. In this way—with a new specially fitted cushion—Sparky would still have his cozy nest, but would not be enclosed. Sparky obviously detested being locked in when he was alone.

Just to make amends for the distress we had caused him, we decided to let him have the run of the flat while we were out the next time. As he had after we'd removed the barriers, Sparky seemingly wanted to reward us for our trust. To our relief and joy, our spunky little terrier hadn't chewed anything other than one of his toys. In fact, aside from the corners of a wooden stepstool he couldn't resist, he's never chewed a thing he shouldn't. Classic objects of puppy-chewing such as slippers and the like didn't entice him, though for a time he never tired of transporting one of John's running shoes from the doormat to the middle of the living room. Never from there back to the doormat. And invariably just *one* shoe; not one then the other. Dress shoes didn't spark his interest either. Nor any of *my* shoes. He seemed much taken with this exercise and indulged in it whether we were there or not. We had great fun watching our industrious little canine toting his trophy about.

Sparky certainly never was aware of how amusing and delightful he was to John and me. Or what a *good* little guy he was! Dogs just aren't that conscious of themselves and the effect they have on people. But if he had *deliberately* set out to charm us, and make us happy, he couldn't have succeeded more brilliantly. Those were great times.

Diet, Exercise and Chemicals

Sparky hadn't always been such a delight. Once—it must have been during the "barrier" episode—I remember crying to John, "Oh, why can't I have a dog who sits next to me like a regular dog?!" Well, if Sparky was too much of a puppy to sit still for very long, he suddenly became willing to pause momentarily and listen to what John or I had to say. He cocked his head from left to right to show he was giving our words serious consideration. I often spoke to him just to watch him cock his head and look at me so earnestly. I learned to put in key words having to do with food or the names of favorite playmates.

Sparky was terrific at recognizing the names of dogs he liked: Leslie, Cabal, François, Gus. When I said "Cabal," Sparky knew I meant the white German shepherd he was crazy about. Leslie was a black cocker spaniel that aroused his interest when I mentioned her. François was a bichon and Gus another Aussie, both of whom lived up the block. All were great pals.

To see them play together on the sidewalk was a treat. Passersby would smile or stop and watch, especially when Cabal was a member of the playgroup. That great white dog would good-naturedly drop into the "play position" to accept Sparky's exuberant attentions.

Sparky also quickly identified food by its given name. When I said "cheese," Sparky knew I wasn't talking about tomatoes. We were feeding him a dry dog food at the time. Persuaded by Mary Jo, we had bought those two huge bags at the pet store in Ann Arbor. It certainly was cheaper there than in New York, as we discovered; however, how long could anyone—dog or not—stand to eat the same stuff day in and day out? One of the books we read maintained that dogs don't mind this relentless monotony in diet. I'm not suggesting that a nutritional diet formulated especially for dogs isn't good for them. Only the mind-numbing sameness of it strikes me as unbearable. Mary Jo had sternly advised us not to give Sparky "people food."

"I don't eat theirs and they don't eat mine!" was her motto. She told us that Jack, one of Mary Jo's older Aussies, sometimes would refuse the kibbles as long as three days, but this didn't sway her into offering anything else. "Don't be seduced by those big eyes," she warned. I guess I was an easy mark for seduction because I let our dog have a little taste of whatever was on the menu for John and me.

Sparky's favorite place (after the park, of course) quickly became the kitchen. After I'd tripped over him once or twice—there's no door to our typically small New York City kitchen—I ordered him to back out and he obeyed. Promptly, too. He wasn't going to obedience class for nothing. Sparky nearly always promptly obeyed a command, then just as promptly resumed the forbidden activity. In this case he would resume one inch at a time.

He even became alert to the rustling of cellophane or similar wrapping containing cookies or other goodies. I often told John I'd never known a dog whose ears didn't perk up on hearing these telltale sounds. At first, Sparky had had no such reaction. But, as usual, he quickly caught on. Soon I had to open such packages when he was away at the park or conked out after returning from there. But being asleep made no difference. He would wake up at the slightest sound of crackling paper and come over to give me "the look." The one Mary Jo had warned against giving in to. Alternately, he would suddenly push a wet nose against my calf, reminding me of a certain family member's existence. Whereupon I reminded the certain family member that he wasn't supposed to *be* in the kitchen. Whereupon he promptly backed out and I gave him a cookie for being so obedient.

I had acquired a certain cachet in Sparky's eyes. At least as long as I was in the kitchen. From this quarter had come roast beef and *sauce béarnaise* (a smidgen only of *béarnaise*—but a smidgen of that sort can be effective). No cook could have wished for a more dedicated apprentice. He would sit at the doorway like a little statue, watching my every move. Our dog was a gourmet. What a discriminating palate! Yes, and pigs can fly. Actually, one couldn't *believe* what he picked up—or tried to pick up—outside. Chicken bones were the least of it. We're talking *vile*, absolutely *vile* objects. Neither John nor I could understand how a dog so well cared for would deign to even *look* at such filthy matter.

Now, with Sparky's lymphoma, we had to be especially vigilant about what he tried to pick up on the street. Anything sharp could prove internally disastrous since the strength of his immune system was lowered by the chemotherapy. Still, he seemed to take it all in stride. On our visit to see Dr. Post on September 13, 2000, John had a near-glowing report tucked in his pocket.

As usual, various pets and their owners occupied the small waiting room that evening. The doctor was generally quite punctual, but this time we had to wait awhile. Since the staff veterinarians were also holding hours at this time, most of the animals weren't cancer patients. A few owners said hello to Sparky. We just smiled back, without saying anything. We always tried to avoid getting into any conversations with them, fearful that someone might ask what was ailing Sparky. Sparky looked so cute to everybody, and so lively—we didn't want to reveal his disease and burst their bubble.

After a short while, Dr. Post appeared and summoned us. "Let's check his weight first," he said. We took Sparky directly to the scale sitting on the floor in the corner of the waiting room. "Nineteen-point-two pounds," he said. "Excellent." Now, the books say Aussies should weigh fourteen to sixteen pounds. At nineteen pounds, he was above the book weight; still, that seemed his natural state. But a cancer patient not losing weight was a *good* sign to Dr. Post. I recall that we had once made an effort to get Sparky's weight down a bit. When Dr. Post saw the results—a full pound less than the last weighing—his face indicated a little concern. "We've been *trying* to get his weight down," John said. Whereupon Dr. Post nodded his head, obviously relieved.

Once in the exam room, John produced the paper he had typed that day on his computer. John had it down to a system by now, dividing the page into three sections: "Report, Concerns, and Questions." This week's "Report" section was the longest. Dr. Post read it as we waited silently for him to finish. The Adriamycin seemed to have no effects on Sparky's behavior at all, the report said. Throughout the week his energy had remained high. His appetite had been excellent; no vomiting. There had been a little diarrhea on Monday, but no panting spells all week. Sparky was craving exercise! This was the most gratifying sign—an active dog, enjoying his walks, enjoying his hour in the park, and enjoying his life.

The report noted that Sparky was losing hair (and quite a lot of hair at that). John and I were never alarmed by Sparky's hair-loss periods. We had expected this side effect—it came with the territory. But John, meticulously thorough, saw fit to mention it anyway.

John really thought that the noni juice was definitely a positive factor. But of course, there's no way one could prove that it was having a beneficial effect—there's hardly any documented evidence that it's worth anything at all. But we followed the noni regimen religiously: two teaspoons of the foul-tasting stuff mixed with tomato or fruit juice three times every day, twenty to thirty minutes before meals. The only times Sparky did not get his noni juice were during his diarrhea episodes.

The section marked "Concerns" was about his recently frequent diarrhea. We were wondering if the diarrhea was a side effect of the chemo or if it was related to his diet. "Most likely it's caused by the chemotherapy," Dr. Post said.

The "Questions" were about the four remaining Prednisone tablets Sparky was to take. John recalled when he had taken Prednisone for his cluster headaches, many years ago. He had been warned not to stop suddenly, but to taper off the dosage. Would this apply to Sparky? The doctor shook his head: "Not necessary."

How had his blood count been?

"Perfect."

The rest of the visit was routine—the physical examination, the blood sample, and lastly, the chemo injection. What chemical was it to be this time? "Vincristine."

This would be Sparky's second time using Vincristine—not his favorite nor ours. We settled our bill with Mary at the front desk—$246 for that evening's visit—and leashed our little bandaged pooch. "Keep positive!" I admonished myself "Keep positive…"

Leaving the doctor's office that evening, while recognizing Sparky's obvious progress, it struck me what a serious business this had become. Such high stakes. I thought back to his early encounters with all sorts of maladies and our overreactions that sometimes bordered on panic. Now it all seemed trivial by comparison, but none of it had seemed trivial at the time.

The first few years in particular, it seems, we were constantly running to the Veterinary Center. For diarrhea we no longer bothered. The routine had become familiar: half an Imodium tablet, withhold food for twenty-four hours, then bland fare such as boiled chicken and rice. Imagine having to withhold food from such a dog for so many hours! Often John and I would go out to a restaurant rather than torment our hungry puppy further by eating in front of him.

Once, I happened to leaf through the medical records from Sparky's puppy days. Horrors I'd forgotten about jumped back into my memory. An ugly growth in his mouth, for instance was one of the most revolting conditions he had developed. How could I have forgotten when the mere recollection of it gives me the creeps? A close second in this revolting series was when he spit up worms.

Our dog, needless to say, had received all the requisite shots. In fact, more than he needed, according to the vet who'd initially checked Sparky out at Westside Veterinary Center. "Breeders often overcompensate," he said on reading the certificate Mary Jo had given us. "I know. I used to be a breeder myself."

Sparky had been well looked after, medically, but he threw up worms anyway. That was in the beginning. Later he turned up with tapeworms. John became very adept at recognizing the signs and would promptly go get the pills to eliminate them. Tapeworms were easier to deal with than diarrhea actually, though equally unpleasant. The veterinarian was mystified that Sparky didn't have fleas, which usually carry the tapeworm eggs. But Sparky somehow remained flealess. Of course, he'd been given anti-flea and tick medicine. But medication hadn't prevented the aforementioned horror.

On another day, Sparky came home with an unsightly rash on his underbelly. Back again to Westside Veterinary Center. The rash required a scraping and day-long observation. Perhaps if Sparky weren't built so close to the ground all of this heartache might have been avoided, I thought. But this was our Sparky and we loved him exactly as he was.

As it happened, the rash episode came with an unforeseen bonus. When he came home from his day-long detention Sparky seemed overjoyed to be back, as if for the first time he recognized our home as *his* home as well. He bounced back and forth from me to John, ran this way and that, his ears back and his little tail vibrating nonstop. Pure joy. How could anyone ever get angry at a dog like that?

His closeness to the ground was also the reason our Aussie hated rain. John bought him a yellow raincoat, which made Sparky look awfully cute, but didn't help. What fell down from above bothered him less than what spattered on his belly from below. He'd dig in his paws, Sparky-style, and refuse to budge. Or he'd head straight for the plaza area that surrounds our high-rise. He knew that there he'd be allowed to run without his leash. For some reason, when he's off the lead he doesn't seem to mind the wetness on the ground. Maybe because he is in control, and won't be forced to walk where he doesn't want to—I'm not sure, but it seems to make perfect sense to *him*.

The plaza is a paved, fenced-in rather large space with built-in stone tables and benches, huge elevated planters with trees and a playground area. The building's ground floor is smaller than those above, creating an overhang around the perimeter, a haven in a downpour. Once taken off the leash, Sparky would run out into the open park as if it weren't raining, fly up onto one of the planters and do his business. This posed a problem for me, as I couldn't climb that high to clean up after him. So I wouldn't take him into the plaza. Instead, I would pick him up when it rained and carry him to the curb. John (perfectly capable of jumping up onto the planters) would take him to the "play," as the plaza area was known to Sparky. Sparky accepted readily that John did things one way and I another, and treated us as distinct individuals. However, once a certain routine had been established with one of us, he insisted that we adhere to it!

Now, our weekly office visits to Dr. Post were becoming part of Sparky's routine—not that he was anxious to adhere to *this* ritual! Half a block away from Animal General he would pull crazily in the other direction. We worked on this problem. The waiting room at Animal General always kept a large cookie jar filled with dog biscuits in the waiting room. When John and Sparky trekked off on their regular outings to Central Park, they would pass Animal General. Often John would tell Sparky, "Let's go see doctor. *Treat!*" Then he would take Sparky into the facility just to get a biscuit. This was to make the place seem less objectionable when Sparky really had to go there. Mary would buzz them in, and at first had a concerned look on her face, thinking that something might be wrong because they had come when there was no appointment. But John explained that they had just come for a treat, and Mary understood that it was just to create a good association about the place in Sparky's mind.

So, on September 20, 2000, when it was time to go to see Dr. Post, John got out Sparky's leash. "Let's go see doctor!" he said, effecting enthusiasm as if it were a spontaneous idea. "Go see doctor, get treat!"

Sparky willingly complied, and the three of us set off for the promised destination. But behind our show of eagerness lurked the ever-present apprehensions about what we might find out there.

Fragility and Strength

John had only a short written report this week, and the only question was about the blood count. How had last week's test come out? Dr. Post simply smiled and said, "Blood count's fine!" John always wanted to know how much collateral damage the chemo was doing to Sparky's system. It was a given that chemotherapy was a less than perfect treatment. John's impression of the process was that all these chemicals were basically poisons. While they attacked the cancer cells, they didn't exactly ignore the rest of the body. The white blood cell count was a good indicator of how the immune system was holding up under the strain. So when Dr. Post said "Fine," John gave a sigh of relief, smiled, and said *"That's* good."

After the usual examination, Dr. Post injected Sparky with Cytoxan. The very name always sounded like a poison to me: "Cy-*toxin.*" But, while I winced inside at the thought of these unnatural foreign substances circulating through Sparky's poor little body, I was abundantly grateful for the magic they performed against the cancer. Still, would they ultimately do the trick? I had cried so many times, thinking about this.

We left the doctor's office that night and walked home slowly. One of the side effects of Cytoxan was that it made Sparky urinate soon after the injection. So we let him poke and sniff, which was fine with him. John was being unusually silent. Finally Sparky peed and we stopped for a moment. John's mind was definitely somewhere else, not an unusual occurrence for him—but now he seemed especially distant.

"What is it? Something wrong?" I asked.

"Oh, I was just thinking. Do you think Sparky'll ever be his old self again, I mean, a normal healthy dog? All these drugs and treatments. I don't know..."

"We'll just have to keep our fingers crossed," I told him. "We're doing all we can." Actually, I think the both of us were going around with our fingers *permanently* crossed.

"Right."

Poor Sparky, I thought. I must have looked like I was getting teary eyed, because John, still holding Sparky's leash, put his arms around me. "It's okay, it's okay. Whatever happens, we'll know we did our best."

"Promise me we'll never let him suffer. No matter what."

"Don't worry, I promise. And if he only lasts another year, we'll give him a good one. At least we'll be able to say we did everything we could."

At that point, Sparky started to express great impatience with our dawdling and tugged on the leash. I broke out of John's arms and looked at Sparky. "I know what *he* wants."

"Dinner!" John cried, and Sparky—in his best sled dog imitation—pulled John all the way home while I trailed behind.

"That dog!" I was thinking, "He's showing us how life should be lived: Just get *on* with it!"

The week that followed was pretty amazing. When we went back to see Dr. Post on September 27th, John could hand the good doctor a glowing report:

> *Sparky's sixth week was superb, the best since his treatment began. His energy seemed boundless, particularly noticeable on his visit to the park on Monday. He ran and scurried up and down stairs and showed great exuberance without tiring. There were no episodes of diarrhea or vomiting this week, and he seemed completely normal (except for the continued hair loss). Urination and bowel movements were unremarkable, consistent with pre-disease patterns. He is tolerating more and more of the Prescription n/d diet, and drinks a full ounce of noni juice first thing every morning (we hear and read good reports on noni—some people attribute it to curing their cancer [!], and we see that it is used by some veterinarians in treating cancer in dogs and cats) and are not unconvinced that it is having a beneficial effect.*

> *Concerns:*

> *Being as Sparky is doing so well in the short term, our thoughts this week have been turning to the future, particularly the long-term effects of the chemotherapy. We're wondering about the frequency and the duration of treatments. At times we feel that perhaps we are buying a year of life while at the same time reducing his chances for much more than that. If a new treatment should turn up, would his body be up to it?*

> *Questions:*

> *We'd like to get a better idea of the effect of chemotherapy, so this is a purely <u>hypothetical</u> question: When diagnosed, Sparky would have survived about eight weeks without treatment. He is currently in full remission. What could be expected if treatment were suspended now?*

Last week you mentioned how bone marrow is damaged by chemotherapy. We hear that a drug called Neupogen can build white blood cells rapidly. Comment?

There is a protocol called DMAC developed at the Ohio State Vet School. We read that this treatment doesn't activate "the multi-drug resistance gene" in cancer cells and has put dogs into full remission in a week's time. Could such a treatment be "parallel tracked" or alternated with the conventional chemo, so that the chemo would not have to be given so frequently?

Since chemo alone promises no cure, what about the combo of Rituxan, the new "monoclonal antibody" with chemo? We read that this combination shows promise in non-Hodgkins lymphoma in human trials.

Sparky is due for an Interceptor tomorrow. OK to take it on schedule?

Finally, for the record, how was Sparky's blood count last week?

Dr. Post, with saintly patience, made no remark about the length of the document. He joked about the noni juice. "Oh, I see," he said. "I'll cure him and you'll say it was the noni juice." Still, he didn't tell us to stop giving the juice. Later, that sentence would stick in our minds. Not the "noni juice" part, but the "I'll cure him" part.

Dr. Post addressed every concern on the list. He said that if treatment were suspended now, Sparky would most likely come out of remission (but not necessarily). On the question of bone marrow damage his answer was that as long as Sparky's blood counts were good, we shouldn't be concerned with bone marrow damage.

It struck me that chemotherapy was a real balancing act. Knowing which drug and how much to give was not a cut and dried procedure. It requires a doctor to know just how much to give based on the current condition of the patient. Since it weakens the immune system while it attacks the cancer cells, the positives and negatives have to be carefully balanced. This takes an oncologist who really knows what he is doing.

Dr. Post addressed the other drugs and protocols in John's list of questions. All were worthy of consideration *if* the chemo failed to keep Sparky in remission. "If it ain't broke—" he advised, leaving it at that. Finally, yes, Sparky could take his "Interceptor" worm pill, and his blood count was fine.

After answering our questions, Dr. Post got down to business. Adriamycin was this week's flavor, and Sparky, as always, lay perfectly still while the doctor pumped the stuff into his veins. It was really amazing. Sparky was such a lively creature. But he gave his utmost cooperation during the procedure. I've seen big macho men—whom you'd expect to be courageous—whimper and whine when they were on the receiving end of some similarly unpleasant treatment from the medical profession. Well, I thought, they could take a lesson from Sparky!

Once back at the apartment, John took the bandage off Sparky's hind leg, and I made his dinner, which he ate voraciously. Maybe, I thought, one day he'll be back to normal. We'll look forward to next summer's vacation. Think positive. I envisioned us all in a car on our way to Vermont. If Sparky is up to it, we'll give him one hell of a good time. We were past the point where traveling with Sparky was a problem. He was now a good, well-behaved animal. We could go and really enjoy ourselves.

I thought about our early experiences with Sparky and cars. Since we didn't own a car, we'd occasionally rent one, most often for summer vacations, but sometimes just for the day. The first time, he was a perfect pest. We had planned to go to Cherrybrook, a popular pet catalog company with a store in New Jersey, about a two-hour trip. The idea was to drive to Cherrybrook, stop, and have a bite at a place with picnic tables or an outdoor seating area where dogs were welcome. We would then browse through the Cherrybrook store and pick up supplies and anything else that might be fun for Sparky. But Sparky wouldn't cooperate. He constantly wiggled out of my lap and crawled over the stick shift to bother John while he was driving, or he'd settle down in the foot well, which was of course dangerous.

Transferred to the back seat, he instantly dove into the foot well there. A kind of harness made especially to keep small dogs in place in a car annoyed him to the point where he nearly choked trying to escape from it. He would sit still only when I, too, went to sit in the back and held him to the seat. What Sparky loved was any stop by the roadside where the smell of food greeted him. So we made a lot of stops. When I think of all the things we've done to accommodate that dog!

People who've never had a dog must think dog owners slightly unbalanced for their excessive devotion to their pooches. Of course, only a similarly "unbalanced" devotee would admit to it. The mother of one of John's students told John she was embarrassed to let on how much she doted on her dog. But there seems to be a built-in partnership between humans and dogs. There is a lovely story set forth by Stanley Coren in *The Intelligence of Dogs* about the god Nagaicho of the Kato Indians of California. When the god Nagaicho created the world, he first erected four great pillars at the corners of the sky to hold it up and to expose the earth...

> *...Then he began a casual stroll around this new world and proceeded to create the things to fill it. The myth specifies how man and woman were made of earth, how the creeks and rivers were made by Nagaicho's dragging feet, how each animal was made and placed in its proper spot in the world— each animal, that is, except the dog. Nowhere in the story is there any mention of Nagaicho, the creator, creating the dog. Rather, when Nagaicho first started on his walk, he took a dog with him: God already had a dog.*
>
> *It seems likely that to the Katos the idea of a human going around without a dog was both unthinkable and unheard of. The dog always was here. After the world was created, the dog simply tagged along behind the creator, sniffing and exploring and listening to Nagaicho's casual comments about his creations: "See how pure the water is in this creek. Would you like to take a drink, my dog, before all the other animals find it?" After a while, the two wandered north together, God and his dog.*

If the Creator himself is so taken with his dog that he makes casual remarks to it about his creations, how can we, mere mortals, be expected to resist the charm of this wonderful animal?

That same year, 1995, Sparky had his first Thanksgiving meal. At home. John served him a bit of everything: turkey, stuffing, sweet potatoes, cranberry sauce, green beans, gravy, the works. Sparky ate slowly, very unlike his Sparky self, as if he knew this was a special meal and needed to be savored. Or perhaps because the fare was unfamiliar and therefore required careful sniffing and tasting before swallowing. As it happened, dinner agreed beautifully with him.

Only a few months prior, on the Fourth of July, his first birthday, Sparky had gotten very ill after eating hot dogs at our balcony barbecue. In retrospect we've come to believe it was yet again the result of something he'd ingested outside rather than the hot dogs. No matter. One had to marvel at his resilience, at how he would bounce back every time after such bouts of illness to reclaim his healthy self.

But what ailed him now surpassed anything that went before. Much as he might want to, much as his valiant nature inclined him to fight back, would he be able to beat such a formidable adversary as cancer? Being in remission was a good thing, but it didn't mean he was out of danger. The treatment caused the cancer to fade quickly, but it could return just as quickly. It was going to take all the strength he could muster.

We were rooting for our little Aussie.

Becoming Civilized

Maybe Sparky would beat this disease by sheer stubbornness. We had noticed Sparky's stubborn streak very early on. If I was walking him and he wanted to take a different route, he'd stop and refuse to budge, forcing me to consider what *he* preferred. Same thing with rain. He didn't want to walk with that wet stuff all around, and suddenly he felt like a 100-pound weight at the end of the leash. For all his peculiarities and willfulness, though, Sparky loved showing off his obedience class training. No, actually that was John, with Sparky as eager participant. Sit! Stay! Down! Wait! Come! Place! John would place a treat in front of him: "Leave it!" And Sparky obeyed and waited for John to give the okay to snatch it up. Those who had witnessed Sparky's early days were amazed at the metamorphosis.

Once we were browsing in a carpet store. John was holding Sparky in his arms because that was the only way the store would admit us. Then one of the salespeople shouted, "That's an Australian terrier!" She told us she had just purchased one—a "red"—and from Mary Jo of all people. The little female Aussie had arrived by plane. When her crate was opened, she immediately jumped up on her new owners, greeting them with great enthusiasm, the saleswoman told us. (Very un-Sparky-like!) The store's no-dog policy was lifted and Sparky and John gave a demonstration of their teamwork to the delight of the applauding staff. Sparky himself looked very pleased. (Anyone who claims that dogs have no expressions obviously never had a dog.)

Outside, Sparky would "heel" and bounce along, looking up at John or me, to the amusement of the construction crew across the street, one member of whom asked me more than once, "Is that a show dog?" Then one day we ran into Phyllis, Sparky's favorite instructor at Follow My Lead. As we were chatting, Sparky, true to form, came up with a chicken bone. "Sparky, drop it," John commanded. Sparky's immediate obedience did Phyllis proud—to say nothing of John and me.

Sparky was such a good dog by nature, willing to indulge our quirks and odd human practices, such as carrying him in to the bathtub to rinse off his dirty feet after every park outing. Upon arriving home, John would put Sparky into a "stay" by the door. This would give John time to remove his coat, put away Sparky's leash, etc. Once in the bathtub, Sparky would extend one paw, then the next, to expedite the ritual. The first time he did that I nearly fell over. But Sparky understood that this was the price exacted for getting free access to the couch, bed, and other contrivances built for humans to sit or lie down on.

He also didn't take long to recognize promises for going out as just that, promises. He wasn't fooled by John's elaborate preparations or announcements—"We're going. We're going."—until he put on his shoes and went to the door. The phone might ring and, Sparky knew, the promise would be forgotten.

One time the phone rang just as they returned. Sparky was left to "stay" by the door until released from the command. After concluding his long conversation, John suddenly remembered that Sparky was still in a "stay." There he was, obediently waiting to be picked up for the feet-washing. A good dog indeed.

John had made the decision, seconded by me, that we wouldn't feed Sparky anything from the table. A begging dog was a nuisance, and we weren't going to cultivate one. This proved a wise choice. After some fits and starts, we settled on three small meals a day for Sparky rather than a single large one. One meal a day, however big, left too long an interval for hunger to build up. The impulse for picking up foreign matter, already overdeveloped in our Aussie, would only grow stronger. Before we ate dinner, I'd give him some dry kibble and, after we were done, some of whatever we ourselves had eaten. In the morning he would get kibble with a little canned dog food for scent and flavor. And at night again just dry kibble. This formula worked extremely well. Sparky accepted it as the norm and didn't beg when we ate, no matter how enticing the fare on the table. He knew he'd get his share and bided the time.

When we took him along to a sidewalk restaurant, however, he became a pest, constantly poking and sniffing and foraging under and around the table. One evening John, exasperated, finally put a newspaper on an empty chair and plunked him onto it. Instantly, miraculously, Sparky morphed into a canine saint. The halo remained in place throughout the meal, so long as he was allowed to partake of it occasionally.

Pesce Pasta, already on our list of preferred restaurants, soared to the number one spot of favorite sidewalk eateries. There were others, but none boasted the advantages of Pesce Pasta: plastic chairs with armrests, perfect for containment, an extra-wide sidewalk plaza, and friendly waiters who liked Sparky, not to mention the manager who himself had a dog named Sparky.

When we went out of town, this was a boon. One motel in Vermont that welcomed dogs had a large canopied outdoor restaurant. It was an attractive space with granite tiles, a bubbling fountain surrounded by greenery and flowers, large round tables, and chairs like Pesce Pasta. Sparky, in his saintly incarnation, drew a lot of comments from the waitress. "He's probably better behaved than some children," I offered. She shot back, "And some adults, I can tell you."

We needn't have worried that this relaxation of rules outside might affect our dog's conduct at home. It didn't. At home, of course, he never sat *at* the table as he did in outdoor cafés. Maybe that was it. In any event, he distinguished between the two and gave us no grief in that respect.

The word *restaurant* became part of our dog's vocabulary. The mere mention of it would set him jumping. Columbia Grammar and Prep School, where John had taught since Sparky was two, was at 93rd Street just off Central Park. Every so often when weather permitted, I would take Sparky to meet John after classes and we'd all walk home through the park together. To get to Columbia Prep one had to pass Pesce Pasta, which Sparky found nearly as exciting as having dinner there.

Perhaps in his doggie mind he fostered the hope that so long as one was *near* Pesce Pasta one might end up there.

Sparky by now had acquired several canine acquaintances in the neighborhood and a few select pals, one of whom was a very special friend named Cavanaugh. This sweet little terrier mix, whose eyes were nearly buried under his charcoal curly fur, would set Sparky speeding in his direction from over a block away, even in the dark. Every time it was a "meet cute" all over again. Our Aussie, who would brazenly snarl at dogs four times his size, would allow Cavanaugh liberties he wouldn't allow any other dog, chiefly Cavanaugh's practice of mounting Sparky's back—which Sparky totally ignored. Cavanaugh came with pals of his own: Roxy, Mushroom, and later, Azul, but Sparky's interest in these was fleeting. It was Cavanaugh he loved best. There was also Hannah—a long-haired Irish Jack Russell—whose cute factor was higher than any dog we'd ever seen. He liked Oscar, a Wheaton, and Brownie, a Chihuahua. Another favorite was Max, a Rottweiler, who was crazy about Sparky. And Gumption, a shepherd mix. Tallulah, a Boston terrier, lived near the edge of Riverside Park. Her owner, Sally, often gardened in front of their brownstone, and Sparky regularly stopped to say "hi." Then there was Judy, a cocker spaniel, and Freckles, a King Charles. Freckles was the name of the dog, but not to Sparky. It wasn't the *dog* who gave him treats. So when I said, "Look, Sparky, it's Freckles!" naturally he shot directly to the lady *with* Freckles.

This speeding-bullet effect was even more in evidence when I would take him to meet John after work. As a rule, I would phone John before Sparky and I left the house. A teachers' meeting might have been called; John might have been detained fixing someone's computer, etc.—any number of obstacles could have cropped up to prevent his joining us. Making that call was like hearing a clarion blast to Sparky. He would spring and prance about, dogging my every step with his nose pushed against my calf. I soon learned to delay such phone calls to the very last moment. Even then he couldn't wait to get out the door and, once outside, would dash forward at top speed, his short little legs racing like pinwheels. I couldn't keep pace and was grateful for any sudden odorous distraction along the way that might detain him long enough for me to catch my breath.

How such a small dog managed such speed never ceased to amaze me. If John was waiting outside the school on the sidewalk, I'd drop the leash and Sparky would sprint toward him, fur flying. Once near John, he'd jump up and down nonstop on all fours to give vent to his joy. It was his own special jump—which never failed to generate smiles from passers-by.

Taking Sparky in a car, though, remained a problem. John, who can't resist a challenge, had been working out an arrangement for the back seat of our rental cars. With the help of foam rubber, pillows, towels, bungee cords and the two separated halves of Sparky's crate, the entire back seat area was transformed into a padded space to confine our ever-busy terrier. Esthetically it was more dust-bowl Oakie than Park Avenue chic, but from a practical perspective it was ideal.

Sparky could sit, lie, stand, and pace while watching the passing scene at window-level. After riding a bit he would settle down in his "tadpole" position to do just that, preferably through the back window. The pleasure quotient during car trips with Sparky rose appreciably, for all three of us.

But now, with Sparky's precarious health and the need to deal with it daily, there would be no thoughts of car trips. Time that we might formerly have spent for recreational activities was mostly used these days for exploring ways to fight Sparky's lymphoma. For this, most journeys were to be taken on the "Information Highway," not the interstates. Lucky for us that John was really good with computers and the Internet. He had always been handy with tools and gadgets, and can be quite inventive. He became interested in computers way back when the best computer you could lay your hands on was a Commodore 64. He has always used computers in his musical work; in fact, he has a whole electronic studio set up in our apartment. When John was diagnosed with prostate cancer in April of 1998, the doctors gave him several distinct choices of treatment, each with its own risks and advantages. The basic four choices were external radiation, radioactive seed implantation, removing the entire prostate, or "watchful waiting." These are typical alternatives, I learned, in prostate cancer cases. In order to find out as much as he could about the disease, John naturally turned to the Internet for information.

He was very systematic, printing out and categorizing relevant material. He finally chose radioactive seed implantation. It was so successful John will be forever grateful that he made this choice—the right one for him. His decision was largely based on computer research. So it was inevitable that he would spend hours at a time at his computer looking for information that might help guide Sparky's treatment. When anything had ever been broken in our home —be it a faucet, a door hinge, or some piece of musical gear—John wouldn't rest until he had fixed it. Sparky would be no exception!

The research was an ongoing thing—hardly a day went by that didn't include an online session. Since the day of Sparky's diagnosis, John had filled two ring-binders with information on lymphoma (animal and human), experimental drugs, and clinical trials. For example, there were pages and pages on a drug called hydrazine sulfate. An excerpt:

> *Hydrazine Sulfate is an anti-cachexia drug which acts to reverse the metabolic processes of debilitation and weight loss in cancer and secondarily acts to stabilize or regress tumors…*

Tests had been done on hydrazine sulphate that showed it was not very effective. However, it was claimed that certain foods work against the efficacy of the drug, and the subjects of the study were allowed to eat these foods, thus invalidating the findings. Oh dear; reading through all this stuff was daunting, even confusing. Such controversy in these pages! So many things to consider! Still, John pursued this information relentlessly. On a typical evening, I might be in bed watching TV, Sparky snuggled up to my side, while John sat at his computer doggedly pursuing information on some new drug, a new clinical trial, whatever. I think what he actually sought was a little hope, in whatever form it might present itself.

He read articles by Judah Folkman, the man who was working on angiogenesis inhibitors. These were drugs that prevented blood vessels from growing. Since tumors need a blood supply to survive, depriving them of blood will kill the tumor. I remember how successful Folkman had been in curing mice with his *angiostatin* and *endostatin*. Human trials were just beginning. We'd have to wait. But would we? *Humans* couldn't legally use these drugs until they were approved. But the laws don't say anything about *dogs*.

On one visit with Dr. Post, John asked if some of the new drugs he had learned about could be made available for Sparky. Even though some of the drugs were as yet unapproved, could Dr. Post, as a veterinary oncologist, get them from the manufacturers? John was particularly attracted to a drug with the cryptic name IM862. He showed Dr. Post his printout from the drug company's web site. The doctor, ever open-minded, took the paper and said he'd look at it.

At Sparky's next visit, Dr. Post surprised us.

"I called the company that makes the IM862. They agreed to send me some."

John's jaw dropped in amazement. "No kidding!!"

"Yep. But understand—so far, the chemo is doing the job. I wouldn't go with something experimental unless Sparky came out of remission."

The implications of this gave us a bit of much-welcomed comfort. If Sparky did have a relapse, at least it wouldn't be hopeless. There would be other things to try. And Sparky wasn't Dr. Post's only patient. It was good to know that he wanted to have as many treatments at his disposal as possible, if not for Sparky, then for another dog. As for all that material—all those pages John had culled over so many weeks—it too became part of the arsenal we would have at the ready, should the worst happen. We continued adding weapon upon weapon to our stockpile, hoping and praying we'd never have to use a single one of them.

A Major Departure

By October of 2000, Sparky looked like a member of a new breed. He had lost so much hair that several people asked us if we had gotten a new dog! I suppose they assumed, knowing his medical condition, that he had died and been replaced. "That's *Sparky*?!" they'd exclaim. Somehow people seemed to be well aware of the effects of chemotherapy on humans but had never given a thought to its effect on dogs. Still, greatly denuded as he was, Sparky retained his high cute factor. He looked very much like the way he once did when getting a bath or swimming. When longer-haired dogs get wet, their coats flatten against their bodies, revealing their actual shapes. Well, that's what our dog resembled. In fact, Kay, our next-door neighbor, opined that he was even cuter in his current state. He looked like a puppy just growing a new coat. He never was actually hairless, as the process of new growth continued alongside the ongoing hair loss, but there was a striking difference in his appearance.

On October 11, we went in for our regular visit with Dr. Post. We could report that he was truly doing well, showing great energy to match his new puppy-like appearance. Dr. Post smiled that twinkling smile he gave when he heard good news.

He checked Sparky's vital signs as usual. First he went over Sparky's body with his hands, stopping to feel for certain things at certain places. "Perfect," he whispered. Then the thermometer and the stethoscope routines. "Perfect," he uttered again and again. These examinations were always tense moments. John and I must have looked visibly relieved to Dr. Post.

Among John's printed questions of the week was the matter of bones. "We've been giving Sparky bones lately, in addition to his regular diet..." one entry began.

Dr. Post put down the list. "No bones!" he admonished. "The chemo lowers his immune system. Bones can splinter and cause internal injuries. We can't risk infections. That's the last thing we want to happen now. We don't need any more problems. *No Bones!!*"

Well. John and I felt properly chastened. "We didn't know. We won't give him any more," I offered, a little sheepishly.

The chemical this time was Vincristine, Sparky's least favorite. I always felt a little trepidation when the flavor-of-the-week was Vincristine. Would Sparky's reaction be as bad as last time? Well, we'll see, I thought, hoping for the best. We thanked Dr. Post and went to the front desk to pay our bill, which came to $246 this time. I took Sparky's leash in order for John to write the check without Sparky yanking at his arm. After John got the receipt from the receptionist, I handed Sparky back to John. Sparky, as usual, pulled John out the door of Animal General with me following close behind.

On the walk home, I thought about the cost of all these treatments. It was hard to believe how much we were spending. Thank God we're in our sixties, I said to myself. John and I had both recently started to receive Social Security. And John was still teaching full time. The additional monthly income just covered Sparky's medical bills—it was like found money. Actually, you might say that the government paid for medical treatments for our dog! I hope they never find out!

But then, there always seemed to be secrets we had to keep regarding our doggie. From the beginning we had been forced to indulge in surreptitious behavior. Keeping him hidden from the powers that be in our apartment building, for example. Sparky cooperated by remaining a quiet puppy. I already mentioned how for the longest time we wondered whether he could bark at all. Considering the no-dog clause in our lease this was, of course, a desirable trait. While we were still laboring under the delusion to paper-train him, Sparky remained in the apartment and no one could have guessed we "harbored" a dog.

When we decided to take him out, though, a strategy had to be devised to keep him out of view as much as possible. The sight of one tiny Chihuahua would trigger a frenzy of activity by the no-dogs contingent in our building. Flyers threatening court action would turn up under doors and be posted on walls. The anti-dog tenants would lodge complaints with management and the landlord and any security guard who came into view. Margaret Hamilton's witch in *The Wizard of Oz* had nothing on *them*.

The hatred is hard to understand in view of the extraordinary things dogs do to help humanity. They guide the blind, tend to the handicapped, and rescue those trapped because of earthquakes or other calamities. They sniff for drugs and bombs, sometimes getting hurt or dying in the process. They protect property and often save lives. Or just plain provide companionship. Is there an animal more devoted to humans than the dog?

All the same, these anti-dog zealots had to be avoided. Luckily, the truly dedicated among them were few, two or three, all female. In a building our size, the chances of encountering one of these in any of our three elevators were slim. It was certain security guards in the lobby we were worried about. At that point we were still bypassing our lobby and exiting the building through the underground, but we couldn't keep doing it three and four times a day. So we decided to enlist the cooperation of those security guards sympathetic to our plight.

Then, one by one, other dogs started showing up on the premises. Some of them with owners who seemed not to care about detection, who blatantly paraded their charges all over the place. This must have occurred slowly, incrementally, but in my memory it seemed to have happened all at once. Suddenly dogs were everywhere, in the elevator, the lobby, even the laundry room. And not only small ones. I remember Cue, a malamute, who was a part of the influx. Sparky and Cue became instant pals.

Anyway, we realized a silent dog such as ours would make a good candidate for staying undetected in the Sherpa bag when the need might arise. Such as while John and I were having dinner out somewhere on our vacation. John had been poring over travel circulars and *Mobil Guide to the Northeast*. After sneaking around so long with Sparky we wanted to stay in a place that accepted dogs. Vermont seemed a good prospect, not too far, and with enough dog-friendly motels to choose from. We enjoyed making our selections and mapping a route where highly rated restaurants were within easy reach. Excellent meals had always been part or our vacation itinerary. We'd rather cut short a stay in favor of including a certain expensive restaurant we wanted to try. But what about Sparky? Leaving our little Aussie, who'd barely gotten used to John and me, alone for what might be hours in a strange room struck us as cruel. This wouldn't do. Not even during the day. Especially not during the day. All it would take was for the cleaning people to open the door and poof!—he'd be gone, escaping to who knows where.

The Sherpa is an ingeniously conceived container. The animal inside sees everything outside through the transparent mesh as clearly as through a window screen, whereas from the outside it looks opaque, unless the bag sits in full sun or glaring artificial light. It's extremely strong and weighs nothing. With the strap slung over the shoulder, it looks for all the world like a piece of luggage filled with something the tourist wouldn't leave behind in the car. Something valuable. (Exactly!)

We decided to conduct a test. Before we sat down to dinner one night, John placed the Sherpa bag near the table, put Sparky inside, gave him a treat, and zipped it closed.

Sparky didn't protest. Didn't make a move or a sound during the entire time John and I were eating. After the meal, John opened the zipper and let Sparky out, and I gave him his customary share of dinner. For a first dry run it was impressive. Several subsequent runs proved equally successful. Here he was, that erstwhile "dog from hell" redeeming himself in spades. Of course the crucial test would have to be administered "in the field." But things certainly looked promising.

Of course, all these little dramas of the past paled in comparison to the huge challenges we were facing now, at the end of the year 2000. To think that, once, our uppermost concerns were sneaking him in and out of our apartment building and hoping he'd remain undetected in his Sherpa bag when we took him into restaurants. To think about how we used to panic over everyday doggie maladies.

As I write this, the report of a genome study has just been published in the newspapers. Dogs have 650 million genes that are identical to those of humans. Gene-wise, I guess you could say that a dog is three-fourths of a human being. Well, doesn't that explain a lot!! I remember reading another survey that reported sixty percent of American dog-owners considered their dogs as they would their children. No wonder. Dogs are our family members, and except for a quarter of their genes, they're humans just like us. Maybe all this had something to do with our absolute commitment to save Sparky at all costs.

Up to October of 2000, we had been going for chemotherapy treatments every week for eight weeks. At this point, the schedule would change to every *two* weeks.

According to the protocol he followed, Dr. Post dropped the Asparaginase (Elspar). I remember saying that I wish it had been the dreaded Vincristine that was dropped, but no such luck. We got to the end of that year with only five treatments, a cycle of three chemicals—Cytoxan, Adriamycin, Vincristine. Looking back, it seemed like all went fairly well. Being there was another story. Would Sparky have a bad reaction to the treatment? Worse, would he come out of remission? As I tried to fall asleep each night, these thoughts—and dozens of similar ones—would jump around in my head, keeping me awake for hours. I started to keep sleeping pills and a glass of water next to the bed. I tried not to resort to sedatives; I didn't want to become dependent on them. But some nights I had to give in—there was no other way.

The calendar flipped over to 2001, and Sparky was still "hangin' in there." All those poisons injected into his little eighteen pounds! Well, actually it turned out that there was much to be said for protocols that relied on a variety of chemicals. John had told me about some cases he read about on the Internet. People reported that their vet "chose Prednisone," or "put our dog on Adriamycin"—and that's all! Who are these veterinarians? Surely, no dog has ever been cured of lymphoma by one single medicine. I wanted to scream loud enough so they all could hear, "Stop!! Get a vet who knows something about chemotherapy!" John and I had come to be firm believers in the "shotgun approach." This is not to imply that you just randomly throw everything at the disease and hope something sticks. But, as yet, a single cure has not been found. Still, a few dogs (five percent) are surviving past two years and beyond. Why? Something must have cured them. As long as we're not sure what it is, I'll stick with the idea of multiple approaches. Besides, the cancerous cells become resistant to the chemicals. That's why, I'm told, animals come out of remission—the chemo just doesn't work any more. Surely, one single type of treatment is not the answer, not yet anyway.

Toward the Christmas holidays, Dr. Post told us on one of our visits that he wanted Sparky to receive special radiation treatments. "I've been generally doing this at the end of the one-year chemotherapy sequence," he explained. "Now I'm thinking that, if I'm getting good results at the end of the cycle, I may get better results by introducing the radiation in the middle of the cycle—after six months of chemo."

He went on to make clear that this would be whole body radiation. Half of the dog's body would be done on the first treatment, and the other half on a second treatment, about a month after the first, so as to give the dog a chance to recover before the second dose was administered.

"Do you do that here?" John asked.

"There's no one in New York who I would trust to do it," he said. "It's not a traditional treatment for lymphoma. I want you to go to Angell Memorial in Boston. I'll give you the phone number there and you can call them and make an appointment." He wrote out the information on a slip of paper and handed it to John. "You'll have to make another appointment a month after the first treatment."

Our dog had been doing well, so far. Might this be the kicker? Hope sprang anew. The next day, John called Boston and made an appointment for the morning of January 4. We'd have to drive there the day before, so that meant an overnight stay. Angell sent us some information in the mail, with driving directions, instructions on preparing the dog, what and when he could eat prior to the radiation, possible after-effects, and a list of accommodations in the area that accepted canines. We noticed that the Howard Johnson's Motor Inn offered special rates for guests with patients at Angell. John called them and reserved a room.

Concluding this business, he hung up, "Well, the room's all set." He finished writing down the reservation information.

"Did you reserve a car yet?"

"No, but I will. I'll do it online; it's easier."

Neither one of us spoke for a few moments. Finally, John looked at me, and gave one of those sigh-like exhalations he makes. He put down his pencil and rested his hand on Sparky, who was on the couch, comfortably nestled against him. "Well, now what?"

"We'll have to wait and see."

Journeys Into the Uncertain

On January 3, 2001, we set out for Boston in our rented car. John by now had gotten very quick at rigging the back seat area, and Sparky appreciated the accommodation. He had come to associate cars with vacations and grassy expanses where he could romp without constraint to his little Aussie heart's content. For Sparky the word "vacation" ranked up there in the glorious company of the word "restaurant." When he saw John behind the wheel, he couldn't wait to hop into the car. (This had made me assume he'd happily pop into any car. But I was quickly disabused of that notion on one occasion when he categorically refused to enter a taxi until after *I'd* stepped in.)

When we arrived at our destination, Sparky would grasp John's leg with his front paws and jump up and down to celebrate. Or run in circles from sheer joy. Sparky liked going to new places: Central Park's botanical garden in full spring regalia; the 79th Street Boat Basin along the wide Hudson River, Lincoln Center Plaza, where the sight of that inviting, wide open space in front of him would inspire him to race forward to a destination known only to him.

This outing, of course, was not a vacation. John and I had been careful not to say the word, nor mention anything about a "doctor" either, which would have elicited the opposite reaction.

We left New York City early, hoping to reach Old Sturbridge Village around noon for the first half of our trip. Even though it was the dead of winter when most shops would be closed in a tourist area, we were certain we would find an eatery of some sort. We would have lunch there, stretch our legs, and let Sparky have a tinkle.

Personally, I wasn't looking forward to a long ride in a car. I'd been seeing a neurologist for pain in my left leg, knee, and foot. The pain intensified whenever I rose from a sitting position, unbearably so at times, to the point where I feared sitting down altogether. Test after test taken with the neurologist—an excellent one, too—proved negative. I had already had several sessions with a chiropractor, seen a podiatrist, an orthopedist, a joint specialist, been given various x-rays and an MRI, all without coming close to a diagnosis. Eventually, a physical therapist would be the first one to mention it might be my hip.

Meanwhile, I was still at the stage where I dreaded sitting down, for fear of what followed when I stood up. Whatever I could possibly accomplish around the house while standing was done in that way. Crossword puzzles, one of my favorite pastimes, were solved—or unsolved—standing at the kitchen counter. While these excruciating episodes lasted, mercifully, only a few minutes, the fear of them was such that I would have done anything to avoid them. The rest of the time there was pain too. It nagged me—it was always there—but it was bearable.

We arrived in Sturbridge Village in good time. Most shops were indeed closed, as we had surmised. After driving around some, we came upon Admiral T. J. O'Brien's, a promising prospect for lunch. The trip thus far had been pleasant. A cold winter day, but the snow, so gleefully anticipated by the weatherman, had not materialized. Sparky was in fine spirits. He looked out the car window as John drove to the far end of the restaurant's large parking area. In summer the lot was probably filled to capacity. Today there were only a few vehicles, mostly pickup trucks, doubtless of local origin. The reason John drove to the extreme end of the near-empty parking lot was so no one would notice Sparky getting into the Sherpa. An empty lot isn't a good place to hide. And Admiral T. J. O'Brien's had an elevated dining room extending from the main building, glassed in on three sides and overlooking the entire parking area. An outdoor deck wrapped around the room, and customers might have easily seen Sparky if the place had been crowded.

Piles of snow were still sitting around the perimeter of the lot. Our dog loved snow and headed straight for it the moment the car door opened. John helped me get up, and we both held our breath, and…there was no excruciating pain. Nothing happened. Was it the bucket seat? Was it a fluke? A lucky break? Whatever the case, I was delighted. So was John. Sparky was too, but for a different reason. Even though the kitchen was way over on the other side of the restaurant, his superior nose had already recognized the place for what it was.

He willingly slid into the Sherpa for, as he knew from experience, savory items could be expected to fill his bowl upon return to the car.

We had our meal with the bag and its secret contents resting under the table. "Good lunch," John said as we returned to the car, "Maybe we can stop here again, on our way home."

"Good idea," I said.

The second lap of our trip was uneventful. After some peculiar twists and turns in Boston's unfamiliar one-way streets, we arrived at the Howard Johnson's. Our room, though, turned out to be a "smoking" room. We weren't crazy about this, but that's the price, I guess, for a room designated for folks with dogs. John and I both stopped smoking in 1983 when I was diagnosed with lung cancer. They caught it early, removed half of my left lung, and that was the end of it, except of course for the recovery, which wasn't overnight. So here we were, three cancer victims in a smoke-smelly room. I hoped that Sparky would beat the disease as John and I had, but our prognoses had been better from the start.

The room had two full beds. John and I each took one and Sparky settled on John's for the night. Before I fell asleep he hopped over onto mine, snuggling against my knees. By morning he had returned to John's. At home Sparky slept between the two of us. Away from home, if the room had separate beds, Sparky selected one of us to sleep with through the night. This time around, he jumped from one to the other, which John and I found endearing.

Our appointment at Angell Memorial was for 9:30 A.M.
We checked out of the Howard Johnson's at 8:00, leaving
plenty of time to get there. Angell Memorial is a huge complex,
bigger than some hospitals for humans. John parked in their
large parking lot and we took Sparky inside to register at the
front desk, after which we settled on a bench in the general
waiting room. Sparky was an instant hit. At this point our dog
looked nothing like his former self. The loss of his abundant
hair and the stubbly new fuzz growing in had turned him into
a different dog. With his new close-cropped hairdo, Sparky
looked adorably puppyish. Gary, Dr. Siegel's assistant, claimed
he was the cutest dog he'd ever seen.

Dr. Siegel led us into her examination room. She smiled
as she set Sparky down on the table. She was a nice-looking
young woman with a gentle manner and voice. "What we'll do
today is administer radiation to half of Sparky's body. Then, in
a few weeks, you'll bring him back and we'll do the other half.
The idea of the radiation is to complement Sparky's
chemotherapy treatments, and kind of give him a leg up on the
situation. While the chemotherapy kills the cancer cells, in time
the body becomes resistant to the chemo, and it fails to remain
effective. What the radiation does is to kill the cells' ability to
reproduce themselves. What we hope to do is close the circle
and extend Sparky's life. The radiation should definitely help.
Of course, Dr. Post has even greater faith in this process—more
conclusive ideas about it being a contributing factor to a
possible cure—"

My heart skipped a beat. John looked stunned. Possible cure?... But we wouldn't indulge in any false hopes. Only time would tell.

Dr. Siegel directed us to a smaller room where people waited while their animals received radiation. After fifteen minutes or so it was our turn. The attendant took Sparky away, and we waited anxiously. I tried to concentrate on a crossword puzzle. John picked up a magazine, then fell into conversation with a man with a golden retriever. So many dogs get cancer! Sooner than I expected, our little guy was back, looking none the worse for the experience. He was hungry—having had no food or water since the previous night—but could we feed him? Dr. Siegel had left instructions at the desk:

Sparky had half body radiation today—We treated his front half (diaphragm forward).

Sparky handled everything well.

Monitor for poor appetite, vomiting, diarrhea and weakness.

Your should see Dr. Post in 2 weeks for bloodwork & chemotherapy.

We can schedule his next half body (back half) in 4 weeks. Please call Gary to schedule a day/time.

Please call if Questions/Problems.

S. Siegel

I headed for the car with Sparky while John stopped at the main desk to pay the bill. Sparky's appetite had definitely not been affected by the morning's events. He made short work of the kibbles I gave him in the parking lot. When John walked out the main entrance and headed toward the car, Sparky rushed to greet him and grabbed his leg to celebrate, nearly causing John to fall over in the process.

Sparky acted normal on the way home. Following our previous idea, we stopped again at Admiral T. J. O'Brien's for lunch. The restaurant's outdoor deck was deserted, but various diners were visible in the sunshine behind the glass. Sparky got inside his Sherpa bag. Once our precious cargo was inside, the bag itself didn't attract attention. However, the bright winter sun was streaming through the window by our table. Its rays went right through the Sherpa's mesh sides. Two ladies having lunch across from us could see our dog plain as day sleeping in his cocoon under the table! To our relief they didn't sound the alarm, but were amused to the point we feared someone would notice. John and I prided ourselves on our foresight with respect to everything to do with Sparky and the Sherpa, but this hadn't happened before. We hurried through our desserts and scooted out of there.

As we drove home I thought about how fortunate we had been with the two women who noticed Sparky in the restaurant. That had not been the only time we'd had cause to worry about others bringing unwanted attention to Sparky. The first time in particular made us nervous wrecks. After all those flawless dry runs at home, a disaster was bound to happen on D-Day. Wasn't it too good to be true? It was the summer of 1996, our very first vacation to Vermont with Sparky. We had yet to discover the Vermonter Motor Inn in Bennington and were en route to Burlington where we had a reservation in an EconoLodge that accepted dogs. We had already made a few stops along the way. Whenever an eatery with outdoor seating came into view—it was our vacation after all—John would put on the brakes and swing off the highway or, if that was not feasible, make the next possible turnaround and double back to it. As soon as Sparky was out of the car, he would jump up and down John's leg to express his approval. If it was this easy to make this little creature happy, how could we not indulge him?

The EconoLodge in Burlington turned out to be well-appointed. There was a pool, a breakfast room for patrons, grassy lawns everywhere, plus a restaurant. After checking in and rinsing off the travel dust, we headed for a scenic route and a likely place to try out our Sherpa trick. After some reconnoitering, we found a casual seafood captain's-table-type place. John parked in the back behind another car and went inside to investigate.

"They have booths." He smiled.

"Perfect," I said.

Sparky matter-of-factly stepped into the bag through the opened side. John handed him a treat before zipping it closed and slinging the bag over his shoulder. One end of the Sherpa was mesh, like the sides, but the other end was solid material. The solid end was facing front. In we went, John making straight for a booth, with me right behind to hide the bag and the smiling host obliviously nodding consent.

It was a roomy booth. John placed Sparky and the Sherpa on the banquette beside him and I sat down across from them. John and I perused the menu, giving each other knowing glances above the card, like two secret agents in a spy movie. A chatty waiter appeared instantly to inquire about our well-being, introduce himself, and describe the specials. We ordered a glass of wine just to be rid of him. But there was no need to panic. Our dog didn't produce a whisper of sound or make a move. We were able to enjoy the wine.

Then, as we were eating, a family—mama, papa and four kids—sat down at the table nearest our booth. One of the children—a little girl barely past the toddler stage—started exploring the area, emitting those screechy, high-pitched sounds that so alarmed Sparky. The mama and papa made only half-hearted attempts to rein her in. I looked in every direction but hers in order to encourage a swift departure, but she was fascinated by our Caesar salad.

"Shall I slip her an anchovy?" John whispered.

She squeaked a few syllables that didn't seem compli-mentary, then screamed as an older sibling dragged her off toward a high chair at the family's table.

Sparky's behavior was exemplary. John and I were the catatonic ones. Then John had to go to the bathroom, another possibility we hadn't thought of, theorizing *I'd* be the one doing that. And Sparky wouldn't fuss if *I* were the one away from the table for a few minutes. I went to sit next to the Sherpa while John was gone and held a soothing hand on the bag, much as John had done during the mini-soprano's visit.

John was back in record time. But all our fears proved unfounded. Sparky simply didn't move. Did he think himself beyond the reach of toddler-types by the confines of the

Sherpa? Was he so confident that John would quickly return that he didn't feel anxious during his momentary absence?

In retrospect, we've found to our relief and delight that Sparky just sleeps and waits for our return to the car—where he knows the morsels in the doggie bag will be his (we always travel with lots of "baggies"). Only once in all the years we've had Sparky did he give us trouble. That was in a restaurant in Yonkers. For some reason he would not lie still. The bag under the table was in constant motion. When the waitress would pass by, we would catch her eye and smile, or make some forced remark in order to deflect her eye from what was going on on the floor. Sparky was even making *noises*—little whining sounds. Just in case, John would imitate the sound and try to incorporate it into a sentence. "*Oh-h...N-n-n-n...*I am so sorry to hear that! *N-n-n...*" We got through that one by the skin of our teeth. This episode occurred three or four years ago, and we've never been able to identify the reason Sparky behaved as he did. John has always maintained it was Yonkers. "Sparky just didn't like Yonkers. It happens."

The summer of 1996 was an unseasonably hot one, especially for New England. Burlington locals and visitors alike made constant references to it. It was just too hot, especially for Sparky. Sparky is a cold-weather dog. The Australian terrier is purported to be an all-weather one, originally bred to ferret out vermin from their burrows in all seasons. But *our* Australian terrier clearly preferred the cold season. Nothing could propel him into hiding faster than the sight of the black woolen doggie coat John insisted he wear when the temperature dipped below 32º F.

Many times we've stood outside, shivering in our hooded down parkas and assorted winter paraphernalia, while Sparky took his time, poking and sniffing, sniffing and poking, impervious to the cold, with or without his coat. He looked so cute in it too, with its large collar standing up behind his head like that of a cape. "Count Sparkula," John had christened him.

Sparky did not, however, handle heat so well. Eighty degrees was fine. Eighty-five tolerable. Ninety and above, his eyes would brim with gentle reproach, as though John and I were personally to blame for it. This accusatory gaze was in full bloom in Burlington. In mid-stroll—even along the lake— he would stop and look up at John as if saying "Oh, papa, you are so big and have such long legs and I am so small and have such short legs, and so much fur besides—even stripped down—how can you let me walk any further in this infernal heat?" And John, invariably responsive to Sparky's pleas, would pick him up and carry him. (Sparky also played this little scene when it rained or when he had exhausted himself playing in the park, for our dog was a quick study, and my husband fell for it each and every time.)

Instead of taking long walks, we took day trips in the car: to state parks, resort areas, the mountains. Vermont is a beautiful state, *vert mont* (in French the "t" is silent) means "green mountain," after all. Unfortunately, dogs are not allowed to swim in the state parks there. We could drive through them and stop and admire the splendid scenery, but this wasn't any fun for Sparky. Then, while driving around, we happened onto a beckoning road, and there it was, a beautiful quarry as big as a small lake. And—were we dreaming?—

people with dogs. Dogs swimming, dogs running, dogs playing ball. What a find!

Sparky was instantly at home. He waited impatiently with me while John quickly changed into his swimsuit in the bushes. Then John picked him up and ran into he water. He lowered Sparky into the water, the dog's legs already paddling before reaching the surface. Sparky immediately swam—to shore. John waded in, retrieved him and ferried him into the water again. Once more, Sparky headed straight for dry land. John tried again and again, but Sparky, whether out three yards or thirty feet, repeatedly swam for shore, shook himself, and waited for John to join him. John called for him, but Sparky stayed put on terra firma. I stood at the water's edge, totally captivated by Sparky's antics. Why Sparky kept swimming to shore I don't know, but it wasn't to be near me (though he made a point of stepping on my bare foot—an affectionate gesture he reserves just for me). Maybe it was because there were too many places he wanted to explore. In fact, in no time, he was clambering up onto a rocky ledge, some distance away from us. We could just see his little body over the top of another high rock formation, about six feet or more above the stony ground level. Suddenly Sparky dropped from sight.

"My god!" John cried and rushed to his rescue. He reached Sparky, who had fallen—or, more likely, jumped—all that way down. John looked down at him, fearing the worst. "Sparky—"

Our terrier calmly looked up at John as if asking, "Something wrong?"

Back again into the water they went. And back again to shore Sparky swam. What a good sport he was, our spunky little Aussie!

How much spunk he (and we!) would have to come up with years later, we had no idea. Not long after his first of the two radiation treatments, we found ourselves back with Dr. Post in Animal General for more chemotherapy. Well, I thought, at least in the second six months of the chemo series the treatments would be spaced further (and progressively even further) apart. On January 17, 2001, Sparky was back on the stainless steel examination table receiving Vincristine through the familiar catheter in a rear leg. The nurse held him down on his side once again, grasping his legs in such a way as to keep him immobile.

Once again, Dr. Post's skilled hands carefully controlled the flow of the scheduled poison. We talked with him briefly about our visit to Boston, how well it went, etc. Our appointment for the second radiation treatment had already been made for a date in February. All the while we spoke, I couldn't help thinking about the next week and what the little terrier might experience in the way of negative side effects.

As it turned out, the combination of the radiation and Vincristine, the drug he least tolerated, indeed took its toll. Three days after the chemo was given, Sparky became so weak he even had trouble walking to his food bowl, a trip usually accomplished by what can only be described as a mad dash. He had no interest in anything; he just seemed to be totally depleted of energy. I checked the note Dr. Siegel had written out for us. "Monitor for poor appetite, vomiting, diarrhea and weakness," she had written. All of the above, I thought. Sparky was experiencing all of these—simultaneously. It was almost too much for one little dog to endure.

His travails reminded me of my own, after my lung cancer operation. To reach the lungs the surgeon had to break several ribs open during the process. After the cancerous portion of the lung had been removed, the ribs were then replaced and left to heal. During my recovery the pain was sometimes so intense I didn't think I could bear it. Sleeping was nearly impossible for weeks after the surgery. The simplest daily tasks, such as bathing or tying my shoe became torturous ordeals. But one tries to go on with one's life—which continues regardless of the difficulties encountered living it. So you keep fighting your way through; the only other choice is to stop living. And here was Sparky, weakened beyond belief, trying to eat his breakfast, jump up on the couch, play with a toy, go for a walk, greet us at the door—when he really wasn't up to any of it.

On our next visit with Dr. Post, February 7, 2001, John had quite a list of unfortunate circumstances to report in his inevitable written account. There seemed to be no end to it—John often had to carry Sparky when making potty trips outside. He folded up paper towels and stuffed them into his pockets along with the usual plastic baggies, to clean the sidewalk. I remember, as John picked him up and headed for the door, those two soulful doggie eyes looking at me, trying to convey his puzzlement at what was happening to him. If dogs get depressed—and I think they do—I believe that's what he was. Yet, he never stopped trying to follow his daily routine—

to live his life as best he could. If dogs can be valiant—and I think they can—he was fighting back for all he was worth.

Sparky is fighting back, I thought, *Sparky is fighting back!*

Fifteen Seconds of Fame

Barely had our Sparky recovered from the bad spell of his previous radiation when we had to return to Boston's Angell Memorial for the second half of his treatment. Our appointment was scheduled for 9:30 A.M., Tuesday, February 20th. This was to accommodate John, who had no classes the day before, Presidents Day and, for reasons I've forgotten, was free on Tuesday as well.

About a week prior to this, we had received a call from the public relations manager at Angell. A crew from the national television show *Extra* planned on doing a piece on animals with cancer. Would we sign a release to let them tape Sparky and us for use on the show? We told them sure.

After John hung up the receiver, he turned to me. "What's 'Extra'?"

"I have no idea," I said.

Our television viewing was mostly limited to news, movies, and a few isolated favorites only vaguely mainstream. We immediately scoured the back of the newspaper and riffled through the TV pages. We found "Extra" listed, but, with no descriptive copy, we were none the wiser. We tuned into the show that evening and got a better idea of what it was: a kind of magazine format, current events and popular features frenetically paced, and with a souped-up sound track to match; lots of whooshing rocket-like sounds punctuating nearly everything.

"Imagine Sparky on TV!" I said.

"A star turn on prime-time! We'll be famous!" John joked, a little sarcastically. But I could tell he was very excited at the prospect.

I didn't dread the long trip in the car as I had the previous time, since the pain I feared I would get after sitting for so long hadn't materialized on that trip. Having discovered that car seats were somehow different, I was less concerned about the agony I'd come to expect when standing up after sitting for any length of time. Also, by then, the opinion of the therapist had been seconded by a medical doctor—the source of the pain was indeed a degenerative hip joint. I would need hip replacement surgery in the near future. Rather than being upset about this, I actually felt reassured. Diagnosis is in itself a great pain reliever.

On the Monday in question John went to pick up our rental car at Enterprise and, after rigging the back up for Sparky, we set out for Boston. I can't recall anything about the weather. There must not have been any snow or ice; that I would remember. As before, we had lunch at Admiral T. J. O'Brien, a stop Sparky appreciated. Also, as before, we stayed at the Howard Johnson in Boston and ate dinner in the hotel restaurant, Sparky sweetly napping in his Sherpa bag under the table.

At Angell Memorial the next morning, we took our little canine patient to the radiation waiting room. Sparky at that point had started to grow an entire new coat of hair. Thick and short, it didn't look anything like his former Aussie coat. But his "cute factor" was higher than ever. One visitor, sitting across from us with her yellow Labrador smiled. "He's a-*dor*-able!" she burst out.

An Angell staff member who was crossing the room noticed Sparky on John's lap. "Cute dog!" He smiled.

"But this isn't the way he really looks!" John replied.

While we were waiting for Sparky's return from the radiation room, the camera crew from *Extra* arrived for our interview. They introduced themselves and began taping while a young woman bombarded us with questions. How old was Sparky? What breed of dog was he? What kind of cancer did he have? Did we expect a cure? Why were we here today? Did we really come all the way from New York City for this particular treatment? Why couldn't that have been provided in New York? How much had we spent on his treatment thus far? Did we drive or fly to Boston?

This went on for about twenty minutes. We answered everything as best we could and they thanked us for the interview and left. When Sparky returned from radiation, the crew was there again, taping Sparky as he ran up to us. Sparky made only a passing acknowledgement of the cameras. As we left the waiting room and headed for the main desk they even taped us paying the bill and leaving the facility.

Once outside, John took Sparky for a little tour of the parking lot. It was cold, but there was no need to urge Sparky back to the car. Once he noticed my putting kibbles in his bowl, there he was, eager for something to eat after his long fast. Just like the last time. But unlike the last time when the meal had had no ill effect on him, Sparky didn't do well at all on the trip home. We hadn't gotten out of Boston when he threw up his breakfast. John stopped the car at the first convenient spot, and we cleaned up the mess and took Sparky out.

We were shocked, since the last time all had gone swimmingly. Sparky had happily eaten, and there had been no adverse consequences. Was it because this time the lower half of his body was radiated? Or was it the car? The movement? Poor little Sparky, he looked terrible. Is there anything more pitiful, or sadder, than a sick animal?

The first half of our return trip was pretty awful. Sparky vomited several more times in the car. We stopped every so often to check on him and take him outside. Our lunch at Admiral T. J. O'Brien wasn't the pleasant adventure it had been the previous three times. We rushed through the meal and raced home. Sparky, however, seemed to recover a bit on the second leg of our trip.

Our little Sparky. He took all these medical doings so well. Much as he disliked the very establishments where said doings were imposed on him—and, boy, was he quick to recognize them as such—he forgave us for causing him all this grief the minute he was outside. For example, he always tried to avoid the corner on which Animal General—where he'd been taken so often—was located. Unfortunately, bribing him with treats had not changed his attitude toward the place. Even if the final destination was Central Park, which he of course loved, he balked if it meant *passing by* Animal General. Walking in the very direction toward that corner had become suspicious to him. If the destination *was* Animal General, when we finally got there he would pull at his leash and rush past the door. Or, to avoid the entrance, he'd cut such a wide arc he'd end up in the street. John often had to pick him up to get him inside the door. Yet, once the ordeal was over with, he casually trotted out the door as if nothing had happened.

Once during a visit with Dr. Post I wondered out loud whether our dog had any idea that we were doing all this for his own good. "He knows," Dr. Post assured me. But did he?

What *did* Sparky think of our constantly subjecting him to these detested experiences? Animals seem to take adversity in stride, as inevitable as everything else that happens to them. This was what *was*. No point in pretending otherwise. It wasn't exactly fun for John and me either. But, truth to tell, Sparky handled it so much better.

Our rendezvous with the doctor on March 14, 2000, was no different. It was already time for Vincristine again. If Sparky had known the cause and effect dynamics of the chemo—most notably Vincristine—and the troubles it created, I'm sure he would not have stayed still for the injection.

Dr. Post asked about Boston, and how the trip went. We told him about the crew for *Extra* and our big interview. I mentioned the vomiting in the car on our way back to New York, and suggested that somebody warn people about feeding their pet right after the radiation and popping into a car with him. John sought a little reassurance that the radiation treatments had been worth it. "Just what does the radiation do, Doctor?"

"It kills the cells' ability to reproduce."

Later I sort of put this all together. Hair cells, I learned, are faster growing than most other cells in the body. Radiation attacks the fastest multiplying cells the hardest. Cancer cells, of course, are fast multiplying, so that's why they are affected more adversely than normal cells. So that's why Sparky lost his hair—hair cells are simply more susceptible to the rays. (I know I'm not using the correct medical terms here, but this is the way I understand it.) Not all dogs, Dr. Post told us, lose their hair. It depends on the type of coat they have.

On the walk home—that one-block journey that had now become so familiar to us—John mused "Perhaps the radiation treatments will make the difference."

"I remember Dr. Post saying that the dogs who'd been given radiation after a year of chemo were still around," I said. "*Still around*," I repeated. As we talked, and Sparky poked and sniffed just about every object bordering the sidewalk, I could feel hope brewing. "If those dogs were helped, then maybe doing the radiation earlier will help even more. Maybe it will stop all those cancer cells—after all, Sparky's *entire body* has now been radiated."

John's face brightened, the way it often does when he gets a new idea. "Maybe the few remaining cancer cells will die of old age with no offspring. He might just make it!"

"That's the spirit!" I smiled and changed the subject by ordering Sparky to leave some particularly obnoxious object he had his nose on, evaluating its edibility. I was afraid to jinx anything by verbalizing any optimistic thoughts. It would be like saying that the pitcher has been throwing a no-hitter in the eighth inning. I wasn't going to go there.

Just then, we ran into our UPS delivery man. He smiled, and John said, "How ya doin'?" The man looked at Sparky, whom he knew from past encounters at our apartment door— encounters that featured the inevitable highly audible greeting Sparky would offer every time the man delivered a package. Detecting that the UPS man was slightly perplexed at Sparky's present silence, John explained: "He only barks at people when they come near the apartment." The man gave a friendly nod indicating he understood. He now knew that when Sparky sounded off at him so ferociously it wasn't to be taken personally.

As I mentioned before, for some time after we got him, Sparky didn't bark at all. Never. Total silence twenty-four/seven. Had we bought a Basenji in Aussie's clothing? Soon, however, we found that this unusual quietude was not going to last. We discovered that indeed he could bark, or howl rather, with the best of them. All it took was one of the neighbors on our floor emerging into the hall at the same time as John or I and Sparky, and the concert would begin. Fortunately for us, they were neighbors who were very well disposed toward Sparky. They'd smile and talk to him, but he would have none of it. He would rebuff these friendly advances with the most head-piercing yowls. At least two among them, dog fanciers both, began to shake their head pityingly at the sight of him, sorry that John and I should be stuck with such a neurotic pooch.

Inside the apartment, Sparky didn't make a peep. Anyone entering, however, was greeted likewise—until the interlopers sat down. If they decided to get up, though, the howling recommenced. And if the visitor happened to be diminutive or—God forbid—a child, the howling intensified beyond endurance. We stopped asking people over. And children were barred altogether until further notice.

This went on for the longest time. It did diminish gradually, imperceptibly almost. Must have, because I can't pinpoint when it ended. Then one day, during these noisy goings on, our doorbell rang and our dog barked. Barked! Not howled. And when John opened the door, Sparky raced for it, to bar the caller's entrance. "You are not welcome here, Sir! This is *my* territory!" he warned the stranger standing on the doormat. Small as he was, Sparky displayed no fear of this gigantic human looming above him. He barked his warning, tail erect, and hind legs planted wide apart on the carpet. Our friend was startled and amused by Sparky's ferocity while John and I were in stitches over this unexpected show of territorial claim. "Good watchdog," I told him and gave him a biscuit. He stopped barking just long enough to eat it, then gave an encore performance.

Once allowed inside, our visitor had the good sense to sit down, which reassured Sparky somewhat. He kept close watch, though, all the same. Since the most direct route to Sparky's affection was definitely through his stomach, we handed our friend a kibble to give our watchful Aussie. Sparky promptly accepted the kibble but did not drop his guard for so slight an offer. He kept a wary eye on him.

From then on Sparky became an excellent watchdog, sounding off with an earsplitting "woo-woo-woo-woo!" at the approach of any stranger. He must have realized at one point that the apartment was his to watch over. It was the den for his "pack," and he strove to protect it. He soon learned that a call on the intercom from the security desk downstairs meant that someone would soon be ringing the apartment doorbell. He treated this event as the inevitable approach of a visitor and started his barking immediately, continuing until the interloper arrived at the door. Even a call from downstairs asking us to come down and pick up a package would trigger Sparky off, even though subsequently no one would show up. John would throw open the door to let Sparky see the empty hall. "Nobody," John would say, introducing a new vocabulary word. Our dog would look around to see for himself. "All right then," he seemed to say, and would usually settle down. A ringing phone didn't elicit a reaction. It was just another noise maker to Sparky, as was a buzzing kitchen timer, a whistling teakettle or a beeping coffeemaker.

Though at first we had doubted that Australian terriers were "excellent watchdogs" as the dog books had claimed, we were now convinced. We slept at night with the utmost assurance that Sparky would sound the alarm if anyone tried to enter the premises.

This, with minor refinements, became Sparky's adopted *modus operandi* whenever someone desired entry. The ferocity of his reception never diminished, but Sparky, being Sparky, quickly expected a "good watchdog" reward. He'd come bounding inside between woo-woo-woos—"Wasn't I great?

Wasn't I great? Where is it?"—crunch-crunch and woo-woo, back to the door.

Little by little he mellowed toward the people on our floor, the women especially. One in particular, an elderly Russian lady, Irena, a gentle soul who adored our dog and cooed to him in Russian, Sparky came to love. We couldn't take him to see her often enough to suit either one of them. She had a generous hand with goodies, sure, but that was only part of it. Others, too, gave him treats. "Bring Sparky," she'd urge whenever she ran into one of us in the hall. Pretty soon we had to refer to her by her last name only. Hearing the first, if only in passing, Sparky would get all excited. Usually I would give her a call to check whether it was convenient for him to come say hello. We would speak French, Irena's second language—mine too as it happened—for she had lived many years in Paris. Sparky may not have understood the words, but he soon knew who was at the other end of the line. Once when I was on the phone with my friend, Jeanine, Sparky suddenly got very excited, bouncing against my leg and making breathy little woofs. I scanned the coffee table for a kibble or some such that might have been left there. Then I got it. I was speaking French. That language—those sounds—he associated with Irena. I told Jeanine what was going on and we switched to English. That calmed him down.

An animal's reaction is so pure. You hand him a treat and he's completely happy. You walk out the door and his anxiety is all-pervading, awaiting your return. All you have to do is walk back in, and he jumps for joy. You talk of going to the park, to the restaurant, to go see Irena, and he springs several feet into the air at the mere suggestion, his face lit up and his tightly packed little body atremble with expectation. As humans, our emotions seem always to be tempered and made complicated by our prized reasoning capabilities. I envy the dog's capacity to experience each emotion to the utmost.

One afternoon, John and I returned from a rather lengthy shopping excursion downtown. We got in the elevator just as Irena did. When the three of us reached our floor and John turned the key in the lock then pushed open the front door, a superkinetic Sparky flew at the three of us, practically doing somersaults at our sight. His favorite humans in the world. He didn't know what or who to jump at next. We couldn't go inside; he wouldn't let us. Inspection of our shopping bags, a priority always, was postponed. At that moment he could only give vent to his joy at seeing us. And people wonder why we love our dogs as we do. Mark Twain once said, "I wish I were half the man my dog thinks I am." That says it all, doesn't it?

No wonder we were doing all this for Sparky. The treatments, the extra care, the worry, the out-of-town trips. If you want to see how much people care for their animals, spend ten minutes in the waiting room of just about any veterinary facility. The faces of the owners we saw in the waiting room at Angell Memorial gave perfect testimony to the unbounded affection that exists between man and dog. The lengths that humans will go to in their attempt to save their animals were profoundly exemplified by these owners of cancer patients. This feeling certainly came through when *Extra* aired its segment on animal cancer.

It was very exciting for us anticipating our "appearance" on *Extra*, scheduled for the evening of January 12, 2001. John and I tried to remember all the things we had said to the interviewer. "Do you think they'll use that part?" John wondered, referring to something we had mentioned.

"Let's hope we didn't blurt out anything too stupid," I told him.

That evening, we tuned into WNBC a little before the show's start. Suddenly a promo for that evening's edition whizzed across the screen. "Tonight: Dogs with cancer on *Extra*—coming up next..."

What a tense moment! The program came on, and the two of us sat riveted before the tube, hushed by the excitement. The first segment was about something else; I have no recollection what. Commercials. Second segment. Again, not ours—some other topic we were not interested in. Then, just before the ensuing commercial break, the words "Dogs with Cancer—next." The commercials that followed were endless, it seemed. Finally, the hostess appeared, glamorously attired, standing in the show-bizzy set with those whooshy sounds and that thumping music fading out behind her as she introduced the segment.

A close-up of a man appeared. For an instant I thought he was John, since he wore glasses and had a moustache. He said something about dogs being our family members. Quick cut to an outdoor shot. Maybe this will be us, outside the hospital, I thought, since they had taken some footage of us there. No, it was a back yard of someone's house. A golden retriever who had contracted cancer in his leg was there with his owner. Dog and owner were next seen entering Angell's main door. Maybe we'll be next, I thought—in the radiation waiting room. Cut to a picture of their impressive radiation machine—"from a hospital for people" the voiceover informed us. Whoosh. Thump. Close-up of Dr. Sheri Siegel, the resident radiologist, explaining (in one sentence) how radiation was used to "complete the circle" of chemotherapy.

Voiceover. Then they showed a dog on the table, receiving treatment. "Is it Sparky?" John wondered aloud. Nope. It was that first dog again. When would we be on? They had told us that we would definitely be included. Where were we?

The point-of-view of the piece was indeed the lengths to which pet owners will go for their pets. I'm not sure if the tone was admiration or mockery—one could take it either way. They then turned to the cost—the amounts that people had willingly spent on their *pets*. Flash close-up of a woman. "About three thousand dollars," she said. Flash close-up of another woman. "Thirty-five hundred." Flash. *It was us!* "Over six thousand," I said—and they cut to the hostess. That was *it*? That was our interview? Whoosh, thump-thump-thump. Wait, there we were again, walking out after Sparky's treatment. Close-up of Sparky for about two seconds. The voiceover mentioned him by name (!), quoting our statement that we had been told to expect him to live only about twelve to fourteen months. Ending on an upbeat note, they showed the owner of the golden, happy with the treatment her dog had received and hoping for a full recovery. End of show.

All in all, the entire piece lasted three minutes.

But, you know?—there were people who saw the program that night who commented on Sparky and how nice it was to see him on TV, as if he had actually been featured in depth. Maybe I'm just too square to follow this fast action style. Maybe everybody else is able to view and digest things at this pace. One lady in our building said she was shocked at how much we had spent. (She actually *caught* that?) If she had only known that six months later the figure would double.

New York's winter snows gave way to the warm winds of spring flowing across the avenues and between the brownstones and high-rises. Every other Wednesday found us in the doctor's office for Sparky's treatments. From February to May, the regimen consisted of Cytoxan, Vincristine, and a new entry on the menu—Mitoxantrone—administered in rotation. Adriamycin was dropped. After each Mitoxantrone injection, Sparky had to take twenty pills by mouth, a new wrinkle. It was generally a good period for him. He remained lively and alert, and suffered no major setbacks.

Unfortunately, because things go well doesn't necessarily mean anxieties lessen. In fact, the opposite sometimes happens. John and I were both aware of the possibility of being lulled into a false sense of security only to be struck with sudden disappointment. The only way to handle the situation was to try to live one day at a time—which sounds easier than it is! We looked at each day as a gift. Sparky was, for the time being, wonderfully normal. We appreciated every moment he was with us. We were grateful for that enjoyment, and we savored it. If, one day, things took a turn for the worse, well, we'd worry about that day when it came. Looking back, I realize that the side effects of the chemotherapy and radiation were in fact sporadic. On balance, most of the time Sparky had been living a good life. For this, our gratitude was boundless. Isn't happiness just a matter of gratitude? And how else can we live *but* gratefully?

In May, after an injection of—what else?—Vincristine, Sparky came down with an extremely bad case of diarrhea. We did all the things we were supposed to do, but there was no stopping it. Day after day, the same thing; we thought we would never get rid of it.

When Sparky first contracted the cancer, he had had this same type of seemingly endless diarrhea. We didn't want to say it, but John and I were both thinking it—this was the first sign of his coming out of remission.

"This doesn't look so good, John."

"You mean the diarrhea? Well, let's not read too much into it. It doesn't necessarily mean—" John didn't finish the sentence.

"Yes, I know," I said, a little weakly.

John gave me a good hug. "It'll be okay; you'll see."

What would happen now? Would the chemo treatments be altered? More and stronger chemicals? How is this battle fought? We had no idea.

We slept badly those nights. Not only because we were both worried sick, but also out of fear that Sparky would have a sudden urge in the middle of the night and we would have to whisk him off the bed. Poor Sparky. The illness lasted for ten days, the longest spell of this sort that he had ever had. At night, John would put his hand on Sparky as we lay in bed and concentrate silently, in some sort of prayerlike trance it seemed. He didn't say a word about this, but it happened several times. Later he told me he was imagining that a powerful healing energy was entering his own body and flowing through his hand into Sparky. He imagined it so intensely that he felt it was really happening.

I remember lying there in the dark, recalling earlier experiences with Sparky and spirituality. Mainly I thought about the Christmases we had had with him.

Our last Christmas season had been an exception—pretty drab this time around, because of Sparky's illness. We had put up a tree, sure, but we always put up a tree. Even those Christmases spent in Pennsylvania with John's mother and the family, when our little tree would just sit there collecting dust in a dark apartment, John couldn't bear not to have one. It wasn't Christmas to him without a tree. In the four decades we've been together, I can recall just two Christmases without a tree, both when John was out of town: once on business in Los Angeles and another when he was on tour with a show.

Over the years we developed a routine that evolved into a tradition we came to look forward to every Christmas Eve. At about dusk, we'd bundle up and go downtown to see the department store window decorations. From Macy's we'd make our way to Altman's on 34th and Fifth Avenue, then up Fifth to Lord and Taylor, Saks, then Rockefeller Center where we'd admire the beautiful angel figures and the gigantic tree.

We would watch the skaters for a bit, then go across the street to St. Patrick's to say a little prayer of thanks. We're neither of us churchgoers—John isn't even Catholic, and I could be considered a lapsed one—but this spiritual stop was a must. There was always a lot to be grateful for—just being together and healthy, for starters. Our final stop would be the Rainbow Grill where we'd linger over a special Christmas drink in that lovely space high above the city.

Finally, we'd head home where our glittering tree and the many colorful packages underneath made the entire apartment look festive. John would light candles and put on Christmas music on the radio or a Manheim Steamroller recording, and we would enjoy our savory *vol-au-vent* pastries. The meal, too, had become part of Christmas Eves. These pastry shells were filled with chicken, mushrooms, and miniature meatballs in a delicious sauce redolent of cream, lemon, and Italian parsley. The dish takes the better part of a day to prepare but, fortunately, needn't be prepared the same day—and the pastries nowadays come courtesy of Pepperidge Farm. Later we'd have champagne or some other celebratory libation and open our presents. Still later we'd watch the midnight mass from Rome (always aired at twelve o'clock our time), during which I could rely upon John to fall asleep.

This, with minor adjustments and a few exceptions for bitter cold or beastly weather, became our Christmas Eve itinerary when we were in town. For instance, when the Rainbow Grill was closed for renovations, we opted for the Algonquin lobby for our customary drink. Once, as I recall, the Hilton lobby. Christmas Day we were flexible, having dinner with friends or whatever, but the Eve belonged to us. And then came Sparky.

His first Christmas with us, he was still a rambunctious puppy. Because of this, we cut our excursion short, imagining no end of mischief he might have caused to the ornaments within his reach, the angels and crèche figures under the tree, not to mention the tree itself. He had shown great curiosity about the decorative additions to our living quarters, poking his nose in boxes and bags as John unpacked them, following my husband's every move while also keeping an eye on my progress in the kitchen. When we saw on our return that everything was just as it had been on our departure, we couldn't believe it. What a good dog! Even a package from John's sister in California that we later discovered contained dog biscuits had been left untouched. What a good dog indeed.

Having ascertained that there was no *need* to cut short our Christmas Eve outings because of our dog, we proceeded to do exactly that—cut our Christmas outings short because of our dog. The idea of his waiting anxiously for us in the foyer by the door while we were having fun just didn't seem right. Besides, the Rainbow Grill wasn't what it had been before being remodeled. And the Algonquin is in a neighborhood nearly deserted on Christmas Eve. And Sparky loved opening presents. (We had always opened our presents on Christmas Eve.) He went at the wrappings and bows with teeth and paws with such relish that we made sure there were several packages under the tree for him to contend with. The last two Christmas Eves before his diagnosis, we dispensed with our little traditional outing altogether and took our good dog to the Blessing of the Animals at Park Presbyterian Church.

It is such a colorful, wonderful service, with all the pews lined with dogs, cats, birds, turtles, hamsters, and their respective owners. A choir sings; there is a homily—just like a service for people. It is quite dignified and even beautiful. At the end, the people and their pets line up and go to the front of the church where the ministers ask each custodian their pet's name, and say a blessing for each individual animal. We felt that these occasions brought us even closer to Sparky because all three of us were brought a little closer to our Creator. Josée, John and Sparky: all three of us were God's creatures—what an important thing to have in common! When the evening's soloist rendered an aria from Handel's *Messiah*, and a few hounds responded with their gentle howling, it actually seemed fitting.

Thinking about all these wonderful holidays, I must have momentarily suspended the apprehensions I was feeling at the time and went off to sleep.

I don't know if it was because of the prayers, the blessings, or what—but our fears about Sparky coming out of remission failed to materialize. His bout with diarrhea evaporated, seemingly overnight. All of a sudden he was a regular dog again. I never thought, in my whole life, that my emotions would one day be dependent on the bowel movements of an animal. I thought I must be just a little crazy.

But I was happy.

Uncharted Waters

On *The Pet Show*, Warren Epstein's weekly radio program, Mr. Epstein once claimed that terriers were very clean dogs. That certainly held true in Sparky's case. Even so, on some occasions for whatever reason—maybe he had drunk an inordinate amount of water or had been in too great a hurry to return home the previous evening—nature would call on Sparky before one of his three scheduled walks. Sometimes neither John nor I was in a position to drop everything and take him out. Maybe it was night, or John was at work and I wasn't dressed. Maybe it was pouring rain. We live on the 27th floor so it wasn't just a matter of opening the back door. Though, and this is my point, I'd open the balcony door and urge him to do his business there.

Our balcony is about five feet by twelve feet, with a solid four-foot high concrete balustrade to ensure privacy, and a concrete floor with a drain. But Sparky refused to soil it no matter how passionately I encouraged him. Yet he knew perfectly well that the balcony was outside. Somehow he considered it part of our living environment. He loved lying in the open doorway and letting the air blow over his face and fur. Located on the northwestern corner of our building and so high above ground, the balcony was practically always windy, so much so that it was impossible to keep plants there.

For Sparky this proved ideal. He demanded the door stay perpetually open. On sweltering days, when the air conditioner was running, or in the depths of winter when we'd rather keep the arctic air out, Sparky would gaze through the glass door with great longing, then turn that longing gaze on me. Needless to say, he would get his way. If only for a spell. Yet he wasn't keen at all about going on the balcony itself unless one of us was out there as well. When a barbecue was in progress, or a pot or dish was cooling off on the picnic table, naturally you couldn't tear him away. We thought this was perhaps the reason he couldn't bring himself to use it as a bathroom.

That changed the day a monstrous winter storm covered our balcony in snow with drifts several feet high in the corners. When John pushed open the door that morning to survey the scene, our terrier dove into the snow like one possessed, scattering the white stuff up and about and tinkling lustily into the drifts. We didn't know what to make of it. Our super-clean Aussie leaving telltale yellow trails all over that blinding white carpet? What was going on?

Once the snow disappeared, our dog's desire to recklessly tinkle likewise disappeared. I scrubbed the concrete floor, hoping to dissipate whatever remaining scents might tempt him to a repeat performance. But, scent or no, he had lost interest in that activity. No snow, no tinkling. When the temperature mellowed enough for the balcony door to remain open, Sparky plopped down contentedly in the doorway as before, sniffing the spring air.

Now it was once again spring. We were looking forward to John's summer break in mid-June. Starting June 27, Sparky's chemo treatments were given even less frequently—monthly now. For him to go for such long periods without any treatment was disconcerting at first. But our worries proved unfounded. Sparky stayed in remission.

We started going back to one of Sparky's favorite destinations, Pesce Pasta, the restaurant with the spacious outdoor dining area. The waiters smiled at Sparky. Some of them knew about his disease and asked how he was doing. "So far, so good," we told them. As was nearly always the case, other diners came up to Sparky and talked to him or commented on his sitting so sweetly and obediently in his chair (on the customary newspaper). But our dog had eyes only for the waiters. *They* were the ones who delivered the goods. Whenever one popped out the door carrying an order, Sparky followed his every step. Until the next one appeared. When one approached our table, he would sit up, unable to contain his excitement. "Sparky, sit!" John would command, and Sparky would obey—but not before getting a glimpse and a whiff of what the waiter set down. He looked so dear, our little Sparky, sitting there so politely between us.

His coat by that time had grown back to almost its former thickness, if not its exact color. The dark "blue" part had come in slightly more brownish. But if the original Sparky wasn't there beside the present one for comparison, it would have been hard to tell the difference. So far, so good indeed. I, however, wasn't doing so well. My hip replacement surgery had been scheduled for April 12, prior to which I'd received a hormonal injection to relieve the pain. Complications too tedious to recount here arose and caused me to postpone the surgery until July. The effects of the injection by then had completely worn off and since another such shot was deemed unwise, I was in pain most of the time. Even so, more painful to me was the postponement, having been bumped from the roster at the eleventh hour after going through a series of pre-op tests and exams; and, having been to the blood bank twice. Now all these time-consuming procedures would have to be done over, including the two blood donations. There's an old World War II song I had learned as a child (in Flemish) that says "everything passes." And the awful time I was having now also came to an end. On July 19 the surgery was at last performed—successfully—and I couldn't have been happier, even though I wasn't exactly nimble. In fact, I could barely make a move on my own. The recovery would take several months, the surgeon had warned.

My hospital stay lasted six days. John visited me twice a day. Before leaving home, he would always call to see if he could bring me anything and to make sure I would be in the room when he arrived. (I was doing a lot of limping back and forth to the therapy room.) On the fourth day, John made his usual call:

"Sparky's really getting worried," he said. "I don't know, babe—he's having a lot of anxiety. I always tell him you're with the 'doctor', but he whines when I leave, and scratches on the door after I'm out of the apartment."

"Oh, I miss him," I said. "Maybe you shouldn't come today. Stay with him."

"No; I'm coming. I've decided to bring Sparky with me."

"But I can't come down to the door to see him." Needless to say, we both were well aware hospitals didn't allow dogs inside.

"I'll put him in the Sherpa and sneak him in. They don't check bags."

"Oh! I'd love to see him! But do you really think—"

"Look. He's in remission, but this anxiety isn't doing him any good.. He's *got* to see you."

"Well," I figured, "if they catch you, all they can do is throw you out."

After an hour or so, John appeared in my hospital room—with the Sherpa slung over his shoulder. He drew the privacy curtain around the bed and let Sparky crawl out onto the foot of the bed. There he came, his tail wagging excitedly. "Hi, Sparky," I said, extending my arms to him.

Just then the nurse came in and immediately opened the curtain. "Not in the *hospital!*" she huffed.

John muttered something about it being just for a minute and left the room pronto with Sparky in the bag. I said something equally sheepish to the nurse, trying to mollify her. John phoned when he got home and said the security guard (apparently alerted by the nurse) had severely scolded him as he rushed past and out into the street. I laughed, and so did John. We both felt good that Sparky had this visit—at least now he knew where I was.

The next day John called to tell me he had rented a special high chair I would need when I returned home, similar to the ones provided for hip patients in the hospital. Once I was home again, seemingly glued to that high contraption of a chair, our Aussie quickly grasped that I was not my usual self, and he seemed honor bound to stay by my side. Sparky didn't consider himself a lapdog but didn't protest, as he was liable to, when John put him on my lap for a bit.

Of course all this meant there wouldn't be a vacation again this year. Sparky probably would have been up for a nice car trip to our favored spot in Bennington, Vermont, but *I* wasn't. I spent the summer in physical therapy.

Fortunately my recovery proceeded apace. Sparky didn't like my cane, so I tried to limp around the house without it. The surgeon, too, urged me to abandon the cane. When I did, sooner than expected, he was pleased. I didn't let on that it was really Sparky who'd led me to discarding it early.

It was too bad about our vacation, but nobody complained that summer. We could go on vacation the next summer—if Sparky made it. There was always that big "if."

Before anyone noticed, it was September, and John began teaching again at Columbia Prep. Sparky was slated to receive his last chemotherapy treatment September 19. John and I were looking forward to that, but not without trepidation. Joy over his staying in remission for one year was undeniable, but there was also the fear of what might happen when he was no longer propped up by treatment. "I feel like a runner heading for the finish line," John said, except that it wouldn't be the finish, only the start of an uncharted journey.

Then on September 11, 2001, our city was forever changed by the unspeakable events of the terrorist attack. Classes at Columbia Prep were suspended when the enormity of what had happened became clear. The extent of the horror was still virtually unimaginable at that point. I remember talking to John on the phone when the rumors that it was indeed terrorism were still unconfirmed. I mean, who could conceive of anything so evil? We were as shocked, saddened, and disoriented as the rest of New York—and the country.

Here we were: I was up and walking, even leaving the house; Sparky had survived a full year in the face of a killer disease; John, his prostate cancer on the wane, had just eagerly started a new school year, and suddenly the bottom dropped out of our lives. Our problems seemed insignificant beside the catastrophic consequences of the victims and their families.

Eight days after the attack, on September 19, we went in for Sparky's last chemotherapy treatment. Walking to Animal General we could still smell the foul smoky air hanging over the city. Even though we lived far uptown, about six miles from the World Trade Center, a haze filled the early evening sky and made it appear as if we were looking through a dirty window. It was a reality that felt unreal. The entire city was stunned, but not stopped. People still went about their business; traffic flowed; elevators went up and down. But it seemed like we were all just going through the motions, following a list of things we had to do, a list we had learned by rote. Something had been taken from us, and its absence left a hollow space.

After a brief spell in the Animal General waiting room, Dr. Post appeared, greeting us with his familiar smile. He beckoned us to follow him into the examination room. We spoke briefly about the disaster, and then the doctor got on with the examination and the treatment. Mitoxantrone: the last injection of poison that Sparky would receive. We were silent, as we always were, while Dr. Post administered the drug. Casual conversation would have been like speaking to a surgeon during an operation; these had always been moments of quiet concentration in that little room, except of course for John's whispers of "Still" in Sparky's ear.

When the delicate part was over, and Sparky's leg was bandaged where the catheter had been, it was okay to speak. "What now?" John ventured. "It's scary that there won't be any more treatments. Is there a greater chance now that Sparky will come out of remission, not getting any more chemo?"

"Actually," replied Dr. Post, "the scariest part was during the treatments. It's a very good sign that he never came out of remission the first year. Most dogs do."

John and I simultaneously grasped the full meaning of his words. It was like an instant revelation.

"The longer a dog stays in remission, the greater the length of time he's expected to survive."

"In other words," John pondered, "the longer he stays in remission, the longer he's likely to stay in remission."

"Exactly," replied the doctor.

"Sort of exponential..."

"Yes."

John was beaming. He smiled at me with a look that asked if I understood what this meant. I did.

"I wanted to ask you," John went on, "just what does 'remission' mean? Does it mean that the cancer might still be there, lying dormant until one day it reveals its ugly head? Or what?"

Dr. Post explained, in his matter-of-fact tone, "Remission means that there is no detectable cancer present in the body."

Sparky had been in remission all that time, and we had just discovered what remission actually was! We were both uplifted; I'm sure Dr. Post could see that in our faces. He wrote out a prescription for the twenty Tribissen tablets Sparky would have to take as a complement to the Mitoxantrone.

"When do we see you next?" I asked.

Dr. Post said that he would like to do monthly checkups for six months, then go to every two months for another half-year. Then every six months. Seeing Dr. Post just *twice a year?* The prospect was heady. Perhaps it would come to pass. We left the office that evening with Sparky bouncing along ("like a king") between us. We were doing a little bouncing ourselves.

"Boy!" I said, "What do you think?"

"'No detectable cancer' he said."

"Looks good, huh?" My feelings were different from any I had experienced the entire previous year. John was no doubt feeling the same way, but he didn't answer. The old jinx thing, I guess.

Later at home, when John took the bandage off Sparky's leg, he paused for a second and looked at Sparky in a way that can only be described as lovingly. He picked him up and gave

him one of the most tender hugs I'd ever seen. "How ya doin',
Sparky?" he asked. It seemed like he was about to cry. But he
didn't.

Poster Boy

The next month was uneventful in regard to Sparky. New York City, stunned by the terrorist attacks, somehow began to get back on its feet, brushing itself off, and getting on with its enormous recovery effort. John began teaching a fresh batch of ninth graders in his "Computer Mastery" classes. One of his extra duties at Columbia Prep was webmaster of the school's web site. I recall the school's telephone system going down on September 11 and remaining so for several days thereafter. The Internet, however, was still up and running. As fate would have it, the entire ninth grade had gone on its annual class trip and was actually out of town—to points north up the Hudson River—when the attacks occurred. Their buses had been scheduled to return to the school on the afternoon of the 11th. School, however, had closed early that day due to the disaster. Parents were frantic. E-mails came in to the website by the dozens. Where were their children? When would they be back? How were they to meet them? All bridges and tunnels in and out of New York had been closed for security reasons. No one knew when they would reopen. John hunkered down at his home computer, answering and forwarding e-mails and posting the latest informational updates on the web site. For an entire day and more, our apartment became a communications center. The kids finally got back the next day, safe and sound. Later, John's web site received hundreds of posted messages from children all around the world, expressing their shock and offering condolences to their American counterparts.

Sparky's life through all of this was, as I say, uneventful—meaning unaffected by the events of our human society. Animals are blessed with this beautiful innocence and detachment from the affairs of mankind. Sparky was an integral member of our family, but we were always aware that his world was not ours. In their book, *The Art of Raising A Puppy*, the monks of New Skeet quote Henry Beston, the naturalist who wrote:

> *...The animals shall not be measured by man. In a world older and more complete than ours, they move finished and complete, gifted with extensions of the senses we have lost or never attained, living by voices we shall never hear. They are not brethren; they are not underlings. They are other nations, caught with ourselves in the net of life and time, fellow prisoners of the splendor and travail of the earth.*

Well, we have been privileged to share our time and space on this planet with Sparky.

October 17, the date of our first monthly follow-up visit with Dr. Post, came around quickly. It seemed strange going into that little room with the stainless steel table without undergoing the injection procedure. No nurse holding our patient down while John quietly chanted "Still...still..." in Sparky's ear. John had no written report to offer. There had been nothing remarkable to write down the past month—

except of course the remarkably good health Sparky had experienced.

The doctor simply examined the dog. Stethoscope, thermometer. The skilled hands felt every inch of Sparky's body.

"Perfect," said Dr. Post, uttering the word almost like a whisper—aspirate consonants, quietly and quickly exploding the word as if he was trying to blow out a candle: "Phhurh-fkt." I can still hear him say it.

The months that followed were golden. We couldn't believe it. The original survival time we had been told to expect was twelve to fourteen months. The end of October marked fourteen months of remission. Then came November, December, January—each cancer-free month extending exponentially the chance of a cancer-free future. Echoing in my mind still is that word uttered by Dr. Post at each monthly checkup, and the way he said it:

"Phhurh-fkt... Phhurh-fkt..."

In February, 2002, Dr. Post completed his examination. The doctor began speaking to us, and John pulled Sparky onto his lap.

"This coming fall, I would like to present Sparky to the Society of Veterinary Oncologists, at their annual conference."

Present? I thought—Does that mean taking Sparky to the meeting?

As he continued, it became clear that what he wanted to do was present Sparky's *case*, not Sparky himself.

"What I'd like you to do is write up Sparky's treatment history from your point of view."

"How long should it be?" asked John.

"Not long. A page or two," he said. "I'm going to present some of my findings at the conference, based on histories of my patients. I'd also like pictures of Sparky, if you have some—before, during, and after treatment."

"No problem," I told him.

John and I wrote up our little synopsis and selected the appropriate photos. God knows we had many "befores" and "afters" to choose from—we took no end of pictures of Sparky. Boxes full. However, there was only one "during"—meaning a short-hair shot—that we could come up with. John, resident family photographer, had been a little superstitious, I think, about taking photos of Sparky looking so strangely stripped of his beautiful coat. I suspect he didn't want such a photo to end up being the last picture ever taken of Sparky. Still, he must have overcome his trepidations one time and snapped our dog atop our bed, in all his sparsely coated non-glory.

We prepared everything and dropped it off at Animal General the next Wednesday for Dr. Post to pick up that evening.

A few days later, we received a phone call from him. "Samantha, the head of the Animal Cancer Foundation wants to feature Sparky in their next monthly newsletter. She'd also like to post the story and pictures on the foundation's website. Would that be okay?"

"Sure!" I said. We were so proud of Sparky's story! "Anything you want."

"I'll scan the photos and e-mail them to her," John volunteered.

"Great," said Dr. Post.

The newsletter came out, and we were delighted to see Sparky there on the Internet a few weeks later. Samantha called us to say that she had received lovely reactions from people who read the piece about our very special little friend. "A lot of people called to say how much they liked that story," she said. "I love it too!" Actually, the reaction to that short article was what inspired us to write this book.

We felt we must be the luckiest dog-owners in the world. All this good fortune. All this attention. Still, one has to give caution its due. I recall emphasizing at the end of that article that we didn't say Sparky had been *cured*. His cancer was "in *remission*—and isn't expected to return."

Xanadu

March flew by. The frequency of Sparky's checkups was reduced to every *two* months. One evening in early April, John and I were watching Burt Wolf's show on television. It's a series that features travelogues and food from regional restaurants. This particular show was about Portland, Maine. After touring Portland's noted restaurants and bakeries, the scene switched slightly south to Cape Elizabeth. What we saw next was a beautiful resort hotel situated right on the ocean: spacious, luxurious apartment suites with full kitchens, lawns, balconies, and an excellent gourmet restaurant on the premises. It was called Inn By The Sea. *"Wow!"* I exclaimed, "Wouldn't that be a great place for our next vacation!"

"Yeah, but a place like that would never accept dogs," John said.

"What a shame."

"Oh well, it was a nice thought."

The next thing we saw was Mr. Wolf sitting with a *tableful* of dogs! Suites came complete with doggie beds, bowls, toys, and treats. *What??!* It had to be too good to be true—or way over our budget. John immediately went to look it up on the Internet and found that, yes, it was expensive, but their higher summer rates didn't start until the end of June. The next morning we booked four days in late June, just before the rates went up.

Later that month, Sparky was invited to be one of the animal Guests of Honor at the annual benefit for the Animal Cancer Foundation at Barbetta's on Restaurant Row. Well! Such attention! Sparky, never at his best among strangers, very small and stuck in the midst of this sea of moving legs, desperately clung to John. The only other face our dog recognized was Dr. Post's, and the sight of that good doctor only propelled Sparky toward the nearest exit.

We aimed for a table and, once safely ensconced on my husband's lap and with me nearby, Sparky relaxed. Then suddenly he recognized someone else and got very excited: a waiter! And this one proved to be the best Sparky had ever met, constantly setting the most aromatic and savory tidbits before us and leaving only to bring still more treats. Sparky now understood why we had come here and why the place was so crowded. The fuss made over him? He decided to tolerate it. "Still in remission!" one guest said.

"Yes," John beamed.

"I read about him in the newsletter. What a success story!" A smiling woman attempted to pet a recoiling Sparky on the head.

"He was cured then?" said a man with her.

"Well, we don't say that," I answered. "We just say that the cancer isn't expected to return." We were very proud and so happy that Sparky was still in remission, but we never had and never would use the word "cured." His cancer was in *remission* and *not expected to return.*

In June, John received notice the school would no longer need his services. This was a blow. He had hoped to remain at Columbia Prep a few more years. My husband loved teaching, and the kids, knowing this, adored him. Also, a few additional years would have made our retirement a bit more secure. But the school was looking at the bottom line. Younger teachers came at half the price. John was well aware of this; he negotiated a severance agreement and looked forward to self-employment again.

Sparky, of course, would miss going with John to his computer lab on Saturdays. John would often go there on weekends to perform maintenance on the server and the workstations. Sparky *owned* that lab—he actually barked when people entered—just as if it were home. Well, all in all, maybe it was a good sign. John's PSA—a prostate cancer indicator—was now very low. Sparky's condition was looking up. My hip was doing fine. The three of us were not to be defeated. Cancer, the World Trade disaster, the loss of a steady income with benefits—whatever—we could handle it. We would be all right. In fact, we were handling things almost as well as Sparky had.

As the date of our departure for Maine grew near, we began assembling a collection of items we didn't want to forget to take with us. A doggie water bowl with a screw-on lid caught Sparky's eye and told him a car was in the offing. Over and above the actual traveling in a car, Sparky knew that at the end of every car trip came something he would like even better than the ride. On the appointed day he trotted happily—plop-

plop-plop—out the door with John "to get the car," as my husband had repeatedly said was the plan.

I could imagine him briskly bouncing along on the sidewalk to the rental office on 83rd Street, which was to serve as his morning walk, then popping into the passenger seat the moment the car door opened as I had seen him do so often before. John would let him ride there beside him for the short ride back to the apartment—a rare treat. He preferred that seat to the back area no matter how comfortable John would make it. As John had done every time. As he did again this perfect June day of 2002.

And perfect it was: a crisp, clear blue-skied summer morning, the kind not often seen in New York. Ideal for the long car ride ahead of us. Cape Elizabeth, Maine, was much farther than Bennington, Vermont. But it was still very early when we took off. John had mapped out our route on the computer as usual, and as usual I was in charge of navigation and tolls.

Sparky was as prepped for this vacation as we were. He gazed out the back window, lying in the "tadpole" position atop his rigged living space, taking in the traffic and scenery. Every so often he attempted to clamber over the barrier (a stiff cushion) John had wedged between the bucket seats and into the front. But I had heard on *The Pet Show* that riding on somebody's lap in the front seat is the worst place for a dog. So I resisted acknowledging his efforts as long as I could, then would let him for just a bit. He would sit contentedly on my lap, looking at John or out the window. But not for long. Predictably, he'd want to sit with John, and would attempt to climb over the stick shift. Okay. Up he went, back over the barrier into his own terrain.

The day was gorgeous and the weather reports on the radio for Maine and environs were equally promising. Not the unusual, muggy ninety-plus degrees type of heat we had endured on Sparky's first New England vacation. This was made-to-order stuff. Ideal indeed.

The remainder of our trip proved equally pleasant. But long. And even longer for Sparky, who made it clear he wanted an end to it. But the ride continued...

"Soon," John told him, trying to make it clear that we were almost there. "Almost vacation! Car almost all done. Sparky wait. Wait a little!"

We had exited the interstate, and John was now negotiating the winding local roads. Just as we were near our final destination, he took a wrong turn. After checking his roadmap, he managed to get us back on course.

"Sparky wait. Al-*most* vacation!"

Finally, there it was. Cape Elizabeth!

Inn By The Sea looked exactly as described on the web site and seen on Burt Wolf's show. John parked the car and Sparky hopped out, then trotted brightly between the two of us to the lobby to check in. There, an attendant promptly handed him a biscuit. The lobby had entrances from both the front and the back. The big doors on this balmy early evening were left wide open, creating a cross current redolent of grass and sea. Sparky sniffed the aroma happily, then jumped on John's leg to tell him as much. We could see into the restaurant. There was no door, only a wide, open entrance. Just inside it stood a white cloth-covered table with information about mealtimes and where one could make a reservation. And, since the dinner hour was approaching, before the entrance stood a cart with serving paraphernalia: bread, butter, condiments, and the like. Bustling to and from this cart was the waiting staff, that species of human so high on Sparky's scale. Could his owners pick a vacation spot or what?! He could barely contain himself.

But, little gentleman that he could be when decorum required, he plop-plopped demurely with John and me down the corridor behind the bellhop and valet cart with our luggage.

Once the bellhop was gone, Sparky ran up and down the halls of our suite, checking out every one of its four rooms, jumping on John's leg between inspections to express his approval. When John opened the porch doors, Sparky leapt out and, seeing the huge lawn, went berserk, rolling in the grass, rushing back to jump at us, racing back again to roll around in the grass some more, celebrating his happiness.

It was wonderful there. We deserved it. *Sparky* deserved it. What a delightful time we had—lobster dinners in our suite, chocolates on our pillows, lots of other dogs for Sparky to meet, beautiful weather. Life was good, even if the future wasn't guaranteed. Even if our troubles were not over. Still, I thought, troubles are never over. But, for now at least, they are in remission—and not expected to return.

THE END

Afterword: If Your Dog Gets Cancer

As of this writing, our little terrier is well into his *fourth year* of complete remission from lymphoma. Why did Sparky survive, when most dogs with lymphoma don't make it past even one year? Was it because he had one of the best oncologists in the country? Or, perhaps, the particular chemotherapy protocol he received? Good genes? Could it have been the experimental whole-body radiation? The fish oil or "noni juice?" The diet?— or was it simply the result of answered prayers?

All I can come up with is "one or more of the above." We simply don't know. There must be other dogs, treated for lymphoma as well as other cancers, with impressive survival times. Why did *they* do so well? As far as I can determine, while there are numerous studies focusing on certain treatments, diets and breeds, there haven't been any studies of the fortunate *dogs* who enjoyed extraordinary extended survivals. That's a pity, because a lot of information could be gleaned by examining the histories, diets, protocols used, and the physical make-up of these exceptional dogs.

Formulating Your Plan

Meanwhile, what can you do, as an owner of a dog stricken with cancer, to maximize the possibility of success? The answer is "everything that might reasonably help." For starters, you have to have the best animal oncologist available to you. That's basic. But I don't think it's enough. You have to attack this thing from every angle, all at once! For example, (and remember, I'm not a doctor—none of this is *medical* advice) I happen to suffer from a certain kind of chronic migraine headache. The pain centers around my left eye, usually starting when I first wake up in the morning. It feels like my left nostril is all closed up. I get a kind of queasy feeling, and feel mildly nauseous. My doctor gave me some pills for headache, butalbital. I tried them, and they helped to dull the pain somewhat, but the headaches and nausea remained. Then I tried taking over-the-counter antihistamines, thinking those clogged nasal passages might be the culprit. Helped somewhat. Then one day I tried inhaling steam, which felt great, but only temporarily. I found that putting a little Vick's VapoRub in my nostril enhanced the effect of the steam. Then I tried applying cold to the area, using one of those little plastic cold packs you keep in the freezer. All to little avail. Each treatment made a dent, but none struck a fatal blow to the headache.

Then, one morning when an attack came, I thought, well, I'll try *everything*. Kind of "shock and awe" the headache. I got up and took *both* the butalbital *and* the antihistamines. Then I inhaled the steam for about ten minutes—with the VapoRub. I followed this with my regular morning shower, focusing the hot stream on the left side of my head. Finally, I got that cold pack out, lay down on the couch and applied it to my left eye. Bingo. The pain receded. Only the nausea remained. After experimenting with olives, Coca-Cola, and several other purported anti-nausea remedies, I finally hit on the one that worked. An ounce of dry sherry turned out to be the ultimate nausea weapon. Now, when I wake with the headache I do the whole routine—from pills to sherry. It works almost every time!

That's what we did with Sparky—the "shotgun" approach. Of course, you can't do *everything*. You can't haphazardly throw in every single treatment you might come across. One has to be selective and use a little common sense. For example, we heard that shark's cartilage was being touted as a real possibility in curing cancer. The theory was, sharks don't get cancer (which actually turned out to be unproven) and there was something present in their cartilage that prevented it. But after investigating further, we rejected this remedy. Too many sources said shark's cartilage was *definitely* useless. No studies to back up its cancer-curing claims.

However, noni juice, another so-called "miracle" treatment for just about every malady you can think of, seemed nonetheless interesting. There were very few scientific studies, lots of anecdotal claims that it cures cancer, but nothing conclusive. One study reported by the American Cancer Society did show that extracts from the noni plant (morinda citrifolia) caused tumors in mice to disappear. So noni was one possibility we took seriously. We figured it would do no harm, checked it out with our oncologist, who had no objection. Noni became part of our "shotgun." Why? Because there was a *reasonable* chance it could be effective. *(More on noni, below.)*

Facing Your Responsibility

You have to be determined that you won't lose your dog until *everything possible* is done for him or her. This means doing extensive research, taking full responsibility for all the decisions involving your pet's health, committing significant financial resources, and not settling for mediocre "standard" doctors or treatment. It might mean traveling out of your way to have him treated at the best facility. It might mean shelling out some serious money for the best oncologist. If you need financial help, ask if your veterinary facility has access to funds for this purpose. *(See "Veterinary Financial Aid Institutions" in the Appendix.)*

Be prepared to spare no effort. And don't let anyone tell you to give up before you've even started! I know of so many owners who, when their dog contracted lymphoma, had him put down as a matter of course. With this particular cancer, tumors can appear quickly, seemingly overnight. It's scary and can seem hopeless—until you inform yourself and commit to serious treatment. A vet might tell you that chemotherapy can only buy you more time, only prolong the inevitable. Well, that might be true, but a lot of dogs survive much longer than their vets "expect" them to. And the time you are buying is most often good time, meaning the dog will feel healthy and active. We were shocked out of our minds when Sparky's diagnosis was confirmed. We know how overwhelming it can be. If you get fatalistic about it, well, you've decided the dog's fate right then and there. I don't know how many times I told people that we were "preparing for the worst, but hoping for the best." I never fully appreciated that cliché until Sparky got cancer.

Finding an Oncologist

When a beloved pet contracts something as serious as cancer, the owner needs to find the best veterinarians and treatments available. Your regular "local vet" might be just the ticket, if he/she is well experienced with treatment of cancer. However, you would most certainly do better by trying to locate the best animal oncologist in your part of the country. Your family veterinarian's recommendations could be a start. If you're near a major veterinary college or veterinary hospital, you're at an advantage. Here's a checklist to help you choose a good oncologist:

- A good success rate?
- Board Certified?
- An excellent veterinary education?
- Experienced with your pet's particular type of cancer?
- Recommended by another patient's owner?
- Recommended by other veterinarians?
- Open to new/experimental treatments and clinical trials?
- Has access to well-equipped veterinary facilities?

Each case, each dog, is different. Your oncologist should be able to adjust his treatments according to your dog's reactions. Don't settle for a doctor who slavishly follows one rigid protocol for all patients. Administering chemotherapy, we found, is as much an art as a science. Some cancers—bone cancer, for example—suggest surgery. Whether to operate or not is often a judgment call. The doctor needs to have good instincts based on lots of experience. Take care! Picking an oncologist is one of the most important decisions you will face. It's "make or break" time!

If you're online and have a favorite search engine, it can be very useful in finding the right veterinarian or animal medical center. For example, you might try a search for "animal oncology." We like to use quote marks when we want to search for the whole expression. If you want to find an oncologist in your city, such as "Boston," you might go to http://www.google.com and enter a search as follows:

```
veterinarian +cancer +boston
```

Note that there's no space *after* the plus (+) sign. Typing all lowercase is fine. This search will find all listed pages with the word "veterinarian." It will then weed out all pages that don't contain the word "cancer." From these it will then eliminate all pages that don't contain the word "Boston." This search yielded 4,470 listings when we last tried it. With a little practice, you'll soon be a master searcher! Which brings us to…

Using the Internet

The Internet is famous for its wealth of information on just about every topic—some excellent, some questionable. Animal oncology is no exception. Carefully evaluate the information you find and always consider the source before accepting it. That said, there is no end of *reputable* sources. But you have to remember that search engines are simply looking for words on a page, and don't distinguish between accurate and untrustworthy information.

Most all major veterinary facilities, foundations, and professional associations have a web site. *(Check out the Appendix.)* You can look up veterinarians and animal care centers in your area. You can find clinical trials for animal cancers, helpful books, survival statistics, recent breakthroughs and much more. Take advantage. If you don't have access to the Internet *find some way to get online*: buy a computer, arrange to use a friend's or one at work, go to your nearest library or walk-in computer facility. Without online capability, there's simply too much you're missing—and it's too important to ignore. Books are great—comprehensive and highly useful—but most become obsolete in one way or another the day after they're published. Changes in medicine move at a rapid pace. The 'Net is the only place that can keep up.

Not to toot our own horn, but a good place to start might be our site at *http://www.SparkyFightsBack.com*. Think of our web site as a companion to this book, beginning where the book leaves off. We're constantly updating it in order to point you toward the latest and best information available. There's a feedback page, and a form where you can e-mail us. We try to answer every e-mail personally. Also, there are links to online "support groups" where you can write or chat with other pet owners having similar experiences.

Making Early Decisions

Early treatment is key. Don't overreact, but don't waste a second if you see possible signs of the disease. With Sparky, we first noticed the swellings under his jaw. There are other places to check for swellings indicating possible lymphoma also: on the back of the hind legs and on the body just behind the crotch at the top of the forelegs. Other types of cancer have their own warning signs *(See the list of cancer's warning signs in the Appendix.)*

Also—and this could be crucial—get a second opinion whenever your dog contracts a serious condition. I just got a call from an acquaintance who lives in Colorado. Her Bernese mountain dog had been diagnosed with a "thyroid problem." Swellings had appeared all over his body. The condition got worse; still her veterinarian continued to treat the dog for thyroid. Tragically, by the time she found out it was cancer, it was too late to treat the dog and it had to be euthanized. A second opinion might have spared the dog's life.

Once your dog is undergoing treatment, keep a journal of your pet's reactions. Take this account with you every time you visit your oncologist, to show him/her what your dog's responses were to each treatment received. This will help the vet choose and adjust future dosages and treatments.

Learning About Treatments

Inform yourself about the available tools used to fight cancer. Here's a start:

Chemotherapy

This is the standard, traditional treatment for canine lympho-ma. It is also used in treating many other types of cancer, often as a supplement to surgery. Basically, chemotherapy is simply the introduction of certain chemicals into the body, either orally or, more commonly, intravenously, with the intention of treating the cancer. Typically, chemotherapy relies on the fact that cancer cells are weaker than, or different from, normal cells. The chemicals attack all the cells, including normal ones—but the cancer cells, being more susceptible, are affected to a greater degree. The term "chemotherapy" can include many different "protocols," or formalized series of procedures and drugs. Most protocols call for the use of multiple chemicals. Several of these protocols have been clinically tested as to their relative effectiveness. The one you're most likely to encounter is the "Wisconsin" protocol. Just to confuse you, there is more than one version of *this* protocol.

I've read notes on the Internet from owners who report that their veterinarian has the dog "on Adriamycin," or some other single chemo. I get furious when I read these accounts! A good protocol calls for *several* chemicals, in a certain, balanced order, given on a certain schedule. I find it preposterous that there are vets putting animals on just one chemical! "Chemo," the cornerstone of traditional treatment and a major part of the "shotgun" of treatments I'm suggesting, is in itself a "shotgun" of several approaches. (Think "shock and awe.")

Chemo alone brings most canine lymphoma victims into remission—quickly, too. The difficult part is *keeping* the dog in remission. The body tends to immunize itself against the chemo, and the treatment becomes no longer effective. That's why chemo (in my opinion) needs *outside help!* And this, I think, is where the rubber meets the road: What can we do to best *support* chemotherapy?

You can expect various side effects to occur after chemotherapy treatments. Certain drugs tend to cause certain side effects, mostly diarrhea, vomiting, weakness and the like. It's beyond the scope of this book to go into each one, but I suggest you have your oncologist explain to you what possible side effects might occur each time a new drug is administered. You can also look them up on the Internet. I often go to *www.WebMD.com* and enter the name of the drug into their search box. The site is for humans, of course, but you'll get a pretty good idea of what to expect, since dogs and people have quite similar reactions to drugs. And remember that the side effects don't always turn up immediately after treatment. They could occur several days or perhaps even weeks after an animal receives the chemotherapy.

Radiation

Our oncologist used full-body radiation on our Australian terrier (given on different halves of the body, each on separate visits). For other cancers, radiation may be used in a more targeted way, on specific areas of the body. Sparky's treatments were given at the "halfway point," six months into a one-year chemo regimen. Radiation has been proven to be effective against many cancers, but there are few firm statistics on lymphoma as yet. A recent study concluded that there was no statistical difference in survival rates among dogs with lymphoma that received radiation and those that did not. Our understanding, though, is that no study has yet been conducted specifically on dogs that received radiation at the *halfway point* in an aggressive chemotherapy series. Remember that studies usually evaluate treatments administered under certain specific conditions and procedures. Their value is often limited.

In short, our opinion is that radiation might help some dogs with lymphoma, and is definitely worth trying. Radiation kills the cells' ability to reproduce. Our personal feeling is that this treatment and the timing of it contributed to Sparky's remaining in remission. Radiation must be administered by a radiologist thoroughly familiar with treating your dog's specific cancer. There will be side effects. Certain types of dogs will lose their coats, others won't. Sparky lost his coat but was never bald, since the new hair grew in while the old was (gradually) falling out. Most all dogs will experience weakness and diarrhea, and perhaps loss of appetite. Your radiologist should inform you about possible side effects. *(See the Appendix for a listing of recognized radiology facilities.)*

Surgery

Some cancers indicate that surgery should be performed. It will be up to you to give the veterinarian the ok to go ahead with any proposed operation. Many factors come into play here. Is surgery the only way to treat the cancer? Are there alternative approaches that might be effective? How will the surgery effect the quality of life of the animal? These can be serious questions, involving tough decisions. The age and strength of your dog, as well as the degree to which the cancer has advanced will be factors to consider. I would certainly get a second, and possibly third, opinion wherever surgery is concerned. You might be convinced that the need for surgery is a "no-brainer." I don't think anything this serious is such a no-brainer that you don't need more than the opinion of one veterinarian.

Also remember that, while surgery may severely curtail the cancer in some cases, you shouldn't abandon other treatments and trust in the surgery alone. *Every* cancer needs a many-pronged approach.

Diet

This is a topic for a whole other book, and, indeed, many books (for humans and animals) have been written on the subject of cancer diets. It's an area that alternative and holistic veterinarians get into more than traditional vets do. However, I found that there are probably as many diets recommended as there are veterinarians. Some go completely vegetarian, others recommend raw meat—it can get bewildering. All I can do here is tell you a few basic things that seemed to work for our dog, and wish you the best. Aside from simply maintaining good nutrition, there are several items I suggest you consider adding to your dog's diet.

Many owners have given fish oil during the chemo treatments, as we did. At least one independent study indicates that fish oil (containing "Omega 3") prolongs remission times in dogs. Going by the yardstick "is there reason to believe it might help?" I'd say yes, load it into the shotgun. We put a teaspoonful in Sparky's bowl every night with his dinner.

We also fed Sparky Hill's cancer diet canned food ("n/d" formula), on the advice of our oncologist. This food has a high fat content, providing balanced nutrition as well. The idea is to "starve" the cancer cells, since cancer cells don't feed on fat. Hill's own studies have shown longer remission times when dogs are on this diet. Again, this sounds like a reasonable candidate for the shotgun.

Noni juice? As you have read in Sparky's narrative, we gave him a tropical "cure-all" juice called "noni." While there have been no human clinical trials on noni and cancer, at least one trial had a positive result, as reported by the American Cancer Society on their web site:

> ... *A group of Hawaiian researchers caused tumors to grow in experimental mice and then investigated the results of treatment using specially prepared injections of noni juice. Mice who received the treatment survived 123% longer than the untreated mice. ...Damnacanthal, a compound removed from the root of the noni plant, may inhibit a chemical process which turns normal cells into cancer cells. They stated that damnacanthal caused cells to return to their normal shape and structure...*

We're not making any claims for noni, but, we think it has a reasonable possibility of helping, despite the commercial hype connected with it. We started giving our 18-pound dog one ounce of pure noni juice twice every day since early in his treatment. It's now nearly four years since his diagnosis, and we still continue the noni every day (only one ounce per day now), mixed with tomato or fruit juice to make it more palatable. In the very beginning, we added just a drop or two to some tomato juice (which Sparky loves), and gradually increased the noni to get him used to it. Our manufacturer recommends that it should be given on an empty stomach (for better absorption), so we're careful not to give Sparky any food starting one hour before the noni and continuing for one hour after.

If you decide to use it, be careful about which brand you choose. There's a great deal of difference in the purity and quality of the juice from one brand to another. Some is reconstituted from concentrate; some is diluted with other ingredients ("to make it more palatable"). You want the straight stuff. The juice is rather expensive ($30-$40 per quart), but a quart should last you a while. And you can have it shipped direct for less. Your local natural foods store or the corner vitamin shop might carry noni, but be careful to read the ingredients before purchasing. A less expensive brand might contain a lot less noni juice.

Clinical Trials and Novel Treatments

New drugs and treatments are coming out all the time. Do some of your own research (See "Research Foundations/ Clinical Trials" in the Appendix). Have the information ready. If your dog comes out of remission (and we hope that never happens), it could come in very handy! There are trials for both animal and human cancers. There are federal laws prohibiting humans from using promising but as yet unapproved drugs (except for enrollees in trials), but there are no such laws prohibiting these drugs from being given to animals! I brought to our oncologist information about a promising new drug being tested at the time. He wrote to the drug company and *they agreed to supply him with the drug for use on animals.* Fortunately, our dog never needed it, but I'm sure that others benefited.

Bone marrow transplants have been performed on dogs with lymphoma. This procedure can be risky, but, if successful, can effect a cure. There is a danger of infection, and the procedure is expensive. But if all else seems to be failing, it is worth considering.

The Spiritual Side

This is such a personal thing. There are some people with great religious faith, some with none at all, and some (most?) who fall somewhere in between. I'm in that third category. But I can offer a few thoughts.

I recall a study made just a few years ago in which an attempt was made to scientifically evaluate the power of prayer. A list of hospital patients, all undergoing angioplasty, was divided equally into two groups. The names and addresses of the first group of patients were given to a panel enlisted to help in the study. Each person in the panel was assigned to one of the patients and agreed to pray for that person every day. The second group of patients was not prayed for. None of the patients were aware of the study or that they were being prayed for. The study found that the patients who were prayed for did markedly better than those who weren't prayed for!

A friend of ours goes to a large church that has a "prayer list" for animals. She put Sparky's name on the list, and he, along with the others on the list, was regularly prayed for. Who is to say that that didn't help?

Of course, Josée and I prayed for Sparky also, each in our own way. We recommend that you pray for your animal, if you are so inclined. If you're not the praying type, it couldn't hurt to ask someone who *is* to pray *for* you!

There is a spiritual approach to healing that is *literally* "hands on." Many believe that we have a healing power in our bodies that can be transmitted through touching. I know this sounds a little crazy, but there are cases that seem to bolster the idea. One such case is described in *Love, Miracles and Animal Healing*, by Allen M. Schoen, D.V.M. He writes about a Doberman named Lady who had bone cancer. Dr. Schoen tells how her owner, Mark, communed with the dog:

> *He would sit quietly at home with Lady on his lap, relaxing on his porch in the early evening. That was a time when there was little or no noise outside, no planes overhead, no shouting children in nearby yards, and few cars on the road in front of the house. During those peaceful moments, Mark would say little, but instead would visualize the area in the dog's leg that was cancerous. Holding Lady on his lap, he would breathe regularly, picture the inside of that leg, and imagine throwing the cancer away…*

Lady improved. Again, who can say if these meditations were a factor? My response: "They couldn't have hurt."

Bottom Line

We *strongly* urge you to explore all possible treatments—including alternative, holistic, nutritional, spiritual and experimental—alongside traditional chemotherapy, surgery and radiation. Investigate clinical trials of new drugs. Coordinate your efforts with your oncologist while not depending on him/her to do it all. Build up a backlog of information, even though you may never have to use all of it. No *single treatment* promises a cure for most cancers! Try everything that looks (a) harmless and (b) hopeful. Stay positive—it's best for you, and it rubs off on the dog. Hope is a powerful force. It can open doors for miracles to pass through.

There are no guarantees. You might give it everything you've got and still not completely succeed. But you *will* have succeeded in this respect: You will know that you did everything you could to keep your dog alive with a good quality of life for as long as possible. You will have succeeded in doing your best!

We wish you all the luck in the world.

—John Clifton

Appendix — Resources

For current updates to the following information, visit
http://www.SparkyFightsBack.com

Animal Cancer Warning Signs

Here's a list of cancer's warning signs, compiled by Dr. Gerald S. Post, a Board-certified specialist in veterinary oncology, and Founder and President of the Animal Cancer Foundation. (Yes, this is the Dr. Post you met in *Sparky Fights Back*.) If you're reading this, chances are that your dog has already been diagnosed. Nevertheless, I think this list should be available everywhere possible, for reference.

The 10 Warning Signs of Cancer
By Dr. Gerald S. Post

Pets have become members of our families and we want to insure that they live the longest and best lives they possibly can. As we have taken better care or our dogs and cats they are indeed living longer; yet despite this, or perhaps because of this, cancer is one of the leading causes of death in pet dogs and cats. Some estimates suggest that greater than 50% of dogs over 10 years old will die of cancer. As a veterinary oncologist, I would like to give pet owners some advice on what things to look for in order to detect cancer in their pets. The earlier you detect cancer the better your chance of effective treatment. Below are 10 warning signs of cancer in both dogs and cats. Please understand that these are just potential warning signs and should not panic you, but prompt a visit to your veterinarian.

1. Swollen lymph nodes—These "glands" are located all throughout the body but are most easily detected behind the jaw or behind the knee. When these lymph nodes are enlarged they can suggest a common form of cancer called lymphoma. A biopsy or cytology of these enlarged lymph nodes can aid in the diagnosis.

2. An enlarging or changing lump—Any lump on a pet that is rapidly growing or changing in texture or shape should have a biopsy. Lumps belong in biopsy jars, not on pets.

3. Abdominal distension—When the "stomach" or belly becomes rapidly enlarged, this may suggest a mass or tumor in the abdomen or it may indicate some bleeding that is occurring in this area. A radiograph or an ultrasound of the abdomen can be very useful.

4. Chronic weight loss—When a pet is losing weight and you have not put your pet on a diet, you should have your pet checked. This sign is not diagnostic for cancer, but can indicate that something is wrong. Many cancer patients have weight loss.

5. Chronic vomiting or diarrhea—Unexplained vomiting or diarrhea should prompt further investigation. Often tumors of the gastrointestinal tract can cause chronic vomiting and/or diarrhea. Radiographs, ultrasound examinations and endoscopy are useful diagnostic tools when this occurs.

6. Unexplained bleeding—Bleeding from the mouth, nose, penis, vagina or gums that is not due to trauma should be examined. Although bleeding disorders do occur in pets, they usually are discovered while pets are young. If unexplained bleeding starts when a pet is old, a thorough search should be undertaken.

7. Cough—A dry, non-productive cough in an older pet should prompt chest radiographs to be taken. This type of cough is the most common sign of lung cancer. Please remember there are many causes of cough in dogs and cats.

8. Lameness—Unexplained lameness especially in large or giant breed dogs is a very common sign of bone cancer. Radiographs of the affected area are useful for detecting cancer of the bone.

9. Straining to urinate—Straining to urinate and blood in the urine usually indicate a common urinary tract infection; if the straining and bleeding are not rapidly controlled with antibiotics or are recurrent, cancer of the bladder may be the underlying cause. Cystoscopy or other techniques that allow a veterinarian to take a biopsy of the bladder are useful and sometimes necessary to establish a definitive diagnosis in these cases.

10. Oral odor—Oral tumors do occur in pets and can cause a pet to change its food preference (*i.e.* from hard to soft

foods) or cause a pet to change the manner in which it chews its food. Many times a foul odor can be detected in pets with oral tumors. A thorough oral examination with radiographs or CT scan, necessitating sedation, is often necessary to determine the cause of the problem.

BOOKS

Healing Pets with Nature's Miracle Cures by Henry Pasternak, DVM. Highlands Veterinary Hospital: 2001.

Help Your Dog Fight Cancer: An Overview of Home Care Options by Laurie Kaplan. JanGen: 2004. *http://www.HelpYourDogFightCancer.com* A pet owner's perspective.

Love, Miracles, and Animal Healing by Allen M. Schoen, DVM. Fireside: 1995. Inspirational and illuminating anecdotes by a noted veterinarian. *http://www.DrSchoen.com*

Pets Living With Cancer: A Pet Owner's Resource by Robin Downing, DVM. American Animal Hospital Association: 2000. A knowledgeable vet translates clinical information into a compact, factual conversation with the reader.

The Illustrated Veterinary Guide by Chris C. Pinney. McGraw-Hill Professional Publishing: 2000. 934 pages, all about animal care.

The Noni Revolution by Rita Elkins. Woodland Publishing: 2002. This tropical juice and what it does.

Veterinary Cancer Therapy Handbook: Chemotherapy, Radiation Therapy, and Surgical Oncology for the Practicing

Veterinarian by Barbara Kitchell, DVM, et al. American Animal Hospital Association: 2000

Why Is Cancer Killing Our Pets? By Deborah Straw. Healing Art Press: 2000. Traditional and non-traditional aspects of prevention and treatment of cancer.

ONLINE RESOURCES

Canines In Crisis

http://www.caninesincrisis.org

[Dog owners share experiences; foods; advice on finding vets, etc.]

Delphi Pet Cancer Forum

http://forums.delphiforums.com/petcancer

[Communicate with fellow owners.]

Perseus Foundation

http://www.perseusfoundation.org

[The Perseus Foundation is a good place to start in your search for answers.]

Hailey's Story

http://www.haileybell.homestead.com

[A Doberman surviving lymphoma after four years. Good advice from the owner.]

ThenSome.com

http://www.thensome.com/petcancer.htm

[A voluminous list of pet cancer links]

Land of Pure Gold

http://landofpuregold.com/cancer.htm

[This page is about cancer in golden retrievers, but offers many links to information applicable to all breeds.]

Living with Canine Lymphoma Clondike's Story, David Kintsfather

http://www.pyrbred.org/lymphoma.html

[Story of a Great Pyrenees with lymphoma.]

Pet Web Library

http://www.marvistavet.com/html/body_the_pet_web_library.html

[Information on most common pet diseases. Each type of cancer listed separately.]

VETERINARY FACILITIES

(A complete listing would be beyond the scope of this book. Using the link below you can find all accredited veterinary facilities in any given area.)

American Animal Hospital Association (AAHA)
http://www.healthypet.com
[Find an accredited animal hospital.]

ONCOLOGIST LOCATORS

Find an Oncologist in Your Area — Perseus Foundation
http://www.perseusfoundation.org/page22.html
[Search by state]

American College of Veterinary Internal Medicine—Enter variables (State, Name, Specialty, etc.)
http://www.acvim.org/Kittleson/search.htm

American Holistic Veterinary Medical Association
http://ahvma.org/referral/index.html

RESEARCH / CLINICAL TRIALS

Animal Cancer Foundation

http://www.acfoundation.org

[Co-sponsor of "Sparky Fights Back" and arguably the best non-profit organization devoted to research to find treatments and cures for cancer in animals. They are also interested in discovering more about similarities in human and animal cancers through their "comparative oncology" program. (Check out the April 2000 Newsletter about Sparky.)]

Animal Cancer Institute

http://www.animalcancerinstitute.com/trials.html

[Organization dedicated to finding causes and cures of cancer.]

Cancer Clinical Trial Links

http://www.cancerlinks.com/trials.html

National Cancer Institute

http://www.cancer.gov/clinicaltrials

OncoNavigator Clinical trials, databases and libraries,

www.kar.net/~onconav/biblie.htm

Veterinary Cancer Society

http://www.vetcancersociety.org

RADIOLOGY FACILITIES

[Facilities with radiology equipment are most often among the major veterinary institutions in their area. This list is therefore also useful in finding facilities with more complete oncology services.]

ALABAMA

Auburn University
Auburn, AL   334-844-5045

ARIZONA

Soutwest Veterinary Oncology
Tucson, AZ   520-888-4498

CALIFORNIA

Special Veterinary Services
Berkley, CA   510-848-1550

University of California at Davis
Davis, CA   530-752-1393

All Care Animal Referral Center
Fountain Valley, CA   800-944-PETS

VCA-Animal Cancer Center
Hermosa Beach, CA   310-318-2436

Cancer Treatment Center
  N. Highlands, CA 916-334-7551

Veterinary Tumor Institute
  Santa Cruz, CA   831-476-5777

All Care Animal Referral Center
  Sherman Oaks, CA   818-244-7977

Veterinary Oncology Specialties
  Pacifica, CA   650-359-9870

VCA-West Los Angeles
  West Los Angeles, CA   310-477-7412

COLORADO

Veterinary Cancer Specialists
  Englewood, CO   303-874-2054

VTH-Colorado State University
  Fort Collins, CO   970-297-4195, Toll Free (877) 427-8838

FLORIDA

Veterinary Radiology Specialists of South Fl.
  Cooper City, FL   954-437-9360

GEORGIA

University of Georgia

Athens, GA   706-542-3221

ILLINOIS

Vet Specialty Center

Buffalo Grove, IL   847-459-7535

Veterinary CT Imaging

Chicago, IL   847-945-9181

University of Illinois

Urbana, IL   217-333-5300

INDIANA

Purdue University Vet Teaching Hospital

West Lafayette, IN   765-494-1107

KANSAS

Kansas State University

Manhattan, KS   785-532-5690

MASSACHUSETTS

Angell Memorial Hospital

Boston, MA   617-541-5136

Tufts University School of Veterinary Medicine
North Grafton, MA   508-839-5395

MARYLAND

VCA-Veterinary Referral Associates
Gaithersburg, MD   310-340-3225

MICHIGAN

Animal Cancer and Imaging Center
Canton, MI   734-459-6040

Michigan State University
East Lansing, MI   612-625-1200

Animal Cancer and Imaging Center
Rochester Hills, MI   248-656-3808

MINNESOTA

University of Minnesota
St. Paul, MN   612-625-1200

MISSOURI

VMTH-University of Missouri
Columbia, MO   573-882-7821

NORTH CAROLINA

North Carolina State University - College of Vet. Med.
Raliegh, NC   919-513-6292

NEW JERSEY

Advanced Veterinary Care
Newburgh, NY   845-569-3070

Red Bank Veterinary Hospital
Red Bank, NJ   732-747-3636

Garden State Veterinary Specialists
Tinton Falls, NJ   732-922-0011

NEW YORK

Veterinary MRI and Radiotherapy Center
Clifton, NY   973-772-9902

Advanced Veterinary Care
Newburgh, NY   845-569-3070

Animal Medical Center
New York (Manhattan), NY   212-838-8100

Veterinary Specialists of Rochester
Rochester, NY   716-271-7815

The Center for Specialized Veterinary Care
Westbury, NY   516-420-0000

OHIO
Veterinary Referral Center
Cleveland, OH   216-831-6789

Radiation Oncology Center at MedVet
Worthington, OH   800-891-9010

PENNSYLVANIA
VH - University of Pennsylvania
Philadelphia, PA   215-898-5448

TENNESSEE
University of Tennessee
Knoxville, TN   865-974-8387

University of Tennessee – College of Veterinary Medicine
Knoxville, TN   423-974-8387

TEXAS
Texas A&M College of Veterinary Medicine
College Station, TX   409-845-9081

Animal Radiology Clinic
   Dallas, TX   972-267-3500

Gulf Coast Veterinary Oncology
   Houston, TX   713-693-1111

VIRGINIA

Regional Veterinary Referral Center
   Springfield, VA   800-569-7070

WASHINGTON

Washington State University
   Pullman, WA   509-335-0754

Veterinary Oncology Services
   Seattle, WA   425-867-5886

WISCONSIN

University of Wisconsin
   Madison, WI   608-263-7600

SASKATCHEWAN (CANADA)

Western College of Veterinary Medicine
   Saskatoon, Saskatchewan, CANADA   306-966-7103

FINANCIAL AID

Animal Cancer Therapy Subsidization Society
>Box 3387
>Spruce Grove, Alberta, CANADA T7X 3A7
>780-479-9361 vetcancer@lycos.com
>[Serving Alberta, Canada]

Help A Pet
>P. O. Box 244
>Hinsdale,, IL 60521
>630-986-9504 *http://www.help-a-pet.org/*

IMOM
>*http://www.imom.org*
>[General Support. Chemotherapy cases are treated specially, but funds are often available.]

PAWS—Pets Are Wonderful Support
>1121 Mission St.
>San Francisco, CA 94103
>415-241-1460 info@pawssf.org *http://www.pawssf.org/*

The Magic Bullet Fund
>*http://www.TheMagicBulletFund.org*
>[This is a new fund co-sponsored by the Perseus Foundation and JanGen Press, intended to finance pet cancer treatments for owners in need of aid.]

United Animal Nations

P.O. Box 188890

Sacramento,, CA 95818

916-429-2457   info@uan.org   *http://www.uan.org*

VETERINARY ASSOCIATIONS

The American Veterinary Medical Association

1931 North Meacham Road Suite 100

Schaumburg, IL 60173

847-925-8070   avmainfo@avma.org   *http://www.avma.org*

Veterinary Cancer Society

P.O. Box 1763

Spring Valley, CA 91979

http://www.vetcancersociety.org

[This is a professional society for veterinarians, but their site offers much Information for the pet owner as well, such as cancer warning signs, news on clinical trials, etc.]

American Holistic Veterinary Medical Association

2218 Old Emmorton Road

Bel Air, MD 21015

410-569-0795   office@ahvma.org   *http://www.ahvma.org*

Printed in the United States
36444LVS00003B/58